Congenital Cytomegalovirus Infection

Gabriele Halwachs-Baumann
Editor

Congenital Cytomegalovirus Infection

Epidemiology, Diagnosis, Therapy

Second Edition

Springer

Editor
Gabriele Halwachs-Baumann
Landeskrankenhaus Steyr
Steyr, Oberösterreich, Austria

ISBN 978-3-319-98769-9 ISBN 978-3-319-98770-5 (eBook)
https://doi.org/10.1007/978-3-319-98770-5

Library of Congress Control Number: 2018960263

This Springer imprint is published by the registered company Springer Nature Switzerland AG
The registered company address is: Gewerbestrasse 11, 6330 Cham, Switzerland

Dedicated to all those people having been congenitally CMV infected because of lack of awareness, lack of diagnostic methods and lack of therapeutic possibilities

Preface

Congenital cytomegalovirus (CMV) infection is the most common intrauterine transmitted viral infection, with a tremendous impact on fetuses and newborns.

In this book, the history of this disease, its pathophysiological background, epidemiology and symptoms, as well as diagnostic and therapeutic strategies are discussed. Starting with an outline of the historical background (Chap. 1—*Long known. Long ignored*), Chaps. 2–5 are dedicated to the topics of virus host interaction for defense and transmission, epidemiology (and the influence of socioeconomic differences), diagnosis, and clinical outcome, respectively. Strategies for disease prevention and therapy are delineated in Chap. 6.

Since economic aspects are gaining more and more importance in health politics, Chap. 7 (written by E. Walter, C. Brennig, and V. Schöllbauer) is dedicated to this issue in the context of congenital CMV infection.

This work is based on the latest scientific findings and written in an understandable manner, allowing persons not working in the field of congenital CMV to also profit from it. Thus, the content is of interest not only to medical doctors, nurses, midwives, and economists, but also to a wider audience, i.e., all those who want to inform themselves about this topic. In this sense, it should not only help toward a better understanding of, but also stimulate further research on, congenital cytomegalovirus infection.

Steyr, Austria
July 2018

Gabriele Halwachs-Baumann

Contents

Long Known, Long Ignored: A Brief History of Cytomegalovirus Research

1

Gabriele Halwachs-Baumann

1.1 Beginnings: 1881–1914

In 1881, the year when president James Garfield was shot, and thereafter Chester A. Arthur was inaugurated as the president of the United States of America, in Göttingen, Germany, Professor Ribbert had to investigate the body of a syphilitic stillborn. At that time Queen Victoria ruled the British Empire. Women of the society had to wear stays and skirts covering their ankles, and it was indecorous for a gynaecologist to see the undraped alvus of a women. The examination of the small body bothered Professor Ribbert. In the kidney he found unusual large cells he could not classify [1]. More than 20 years later, in 1904, the two physicians Jesionek and Kiolemenoglou from the Royal Dermatological Hospital in Munich published a case study about 'Findings of protozoan like structures in the organs of an inherited infected luetic fetus'. They wrote that they had investigated almost all organs of the fetus, and in five of them, they found besides changes due to the infection with *Treponema pallidum* the causative organism for syphilis, idiosyncratic cellular formations, whose interpretation made great difficulties. The organs, which showed these peculiar changes, were the two kidneys, the two lungs and the liver, where clusters of 10–40 'elements' were observed. These 'elements' were 20 to 30 μm in diameter, the nuclei were large and eccentrically placed and each contained a 'central nuclear body' surrounded by two zones, a darker inner zone and a clear outer zone, which could be clearly differentiated. This accurate depiction of histological changes, taking more than two pages, is one of the most remarkable examples of exact observations in natural science [2]. Although the authors could not interpret their findings correctly, they described the 'owl eye cells', typical changes in cytomegalovirus infection, which were used as a diagnostic tool until recently.

G. Halwachs-Baumann (✉)
Department of Laboratory Medicine, Regional Hospital Steyr, Steyr, Austria
e-mail: gabriele.baumann@gespag.at

G. Halwachs-Baumann (ed.), *Congenital Cytomegalovirus Infection*,
https://doi.org/10.1007/978-3-319-98770-5_1

One has to keep in mind 100 years ago, to take a 'virus' as pathogenic agents was not granted. Only a few years before, between 1886 and 1898, the first evidence for the existence of pathogens, smaller than bacteria, was provided. Adolf Mayer from the Netherlands showed in 1882 the transmission of the mosaic illness to healthy tobacco plants by inoculating them with the sap of diseased plants. In 1892 the Russian biologist Dimitri I. Iwanowsky showed that this illness is also transmitted even when the sap was filtered by a so-called Chamberland filter, which holds off particles from the size of bacteria. M. W. Beijerinck, a Dutch soil microbiologist, confirmed Ivanowsky's observations and further showed that the infectivity of sap remained constant during serial infections of plants, providing evidence that the agent could not be a toxin, since it was able to replicate itself in living organisms [3]. In 1898 Friedrich Löffler and Paul Frosch, both students of Robert Koch, described the cause of the foot-and-mouth disease to be a particle, smaller than a bacteria, and not a liquid. They made serial transmission of filtered vesicle from diseased animals and concluded if the cause of the foot-and-mouth disease was toxin-based, then after several animal-to-animal transmissions, the original material would be so diluted that only '1:2 ½ trillion' of the starting substance would remain. 'A toxic effect of that nature would be unbelievable' they concluded. So the causative agents must be capable of reproducing itself [3–5]. In his 1899 published paper, 'a *contagium vivum fluidum* as the cause of the mosaic disease of tobacco leaves' Beijerinck used first the term 'virus' for the described infectious agents [6]. 'Virus' from the Latin word for 'poisson', first used by Aulus Cornelius Celsus (25 B.C.–about 50 AD) for the saliva of rabid dogs, became now the term for the small infectious particles, which are not bacteria but can reproduce themselves in living organisms.

So one has to excuse Jesionek and Kiolemenoglou for their assumption that the structures they found are due to protozoans, concretely *Gregarinida*, as they wrote. And Ribbert, who published his observations after he read the paper of Jesionek and Kiolemenoglou, subscribed to their view, although in the last sentence of his paper he wrote 'the value of my memorandum is mainly, by compounding the impression of those both authors, to request further investigations'. These investigations were done, and substantial difference of opinion existed among the various observers. Amoebas, coccidian and sporozoa were regarded as the source and nature of these unusual cellular formations [7]. In 1914 Smith and Weidman described similar findings and gave the name *Endameba mortinatalium* to the structures.

1.2 Between the Wars: 1914–1930

The scientific investigations in this field were adjourned by the First World War, which changed the political, social and economic structure not only of Europe but of the majority of the world. It lasted until 1921, when Ernest W. Goodpasture, at that time assistant professor at the Department of Pathology and Cancer Commission of Harvard University and better known as the first who described a rare case characterized by glomerulonephritis and haemorrhaging of the lung (Goodpasture syndrome), in cooperation with his colleague Fritz B. Talbot, gave the observed 'protozoan-like' changes a name, by writing that '. . .it seems advisable to identify the condition with a descriptive name, and we would suggest, that it be called cytomegalia infantum'. [8] Besides this nomenclature, valid until now, they made in this paper another remarkable assumption, when they wrote that the observed cellular alterations in 'cytomegalia infantum' are similar to the skin lesions in varicella described by Tyzzer 1906 [9] and might be therefore due to the indirect effect of a similar agent on the cell. It is remarkable that Tyzzer, who was sent to the Philippines in 1904 to study the susceptibility of monkeys to smallpox (at that time varicella and variola were thought to be the minor and the major form of the same illness caused by a protozoan parasite), could study the evolution of cutaneous lesions by histopathologic examination of serial biopsies in 38 subjects, infected with varicella during an outbreak of this disease in Bilibid Prison. In the summary of his report he wrote that '. . .no important evidence has been found in favour of the hypothesis that they (the inclusions) are parasitic organisms'. So, looking back to the paper of Tyzzer, Goodpasture and Talbot were the first who supposed that the cytomegalic changes are not due to protozoan, and as it was shown later on, both infectious diseases (varicella and cytomegalia) are caused by virus of the same family.

In the same year (1921), when Goodpasture and Talbot published their paper, Benjamin Lipschütz, an Austrian dermatologist and bacteriologist, reported that similar inclusions were associated with lesions in humans and rabbits infected with herpes simplex. He maintained that the bodies or structures seen within the nucleus represent a specific reaction of the cells to a living virus. The bodies are not considered to be masses of parasites but are held to represent reaction products, associated with which is the virus, he postulated [10]. This conception of Lipschütz was not universally accepted, however. A. Luger and E. Lauda, both scientists working at the University Clinics for Internal Medicine in Vienna at the same time as Lipschütz, presumed that the 'inclusion bodies' are the result of a non-specific type of nuclear degeneration, which these authors call 'oxychromatic degeneration' [11]. All these papers were known by Rufus Cole, who became later on the first director of the Hospital of the Rockefeller Institute for Medical Research, and Ann Gayler Kuttner, who wrote her thesis for the PhD on bacteriophage phenomena, a subject which was very popular at that time ("Arrowsmith" a novel published 1925 by Sinclair Lewis, the first American to be awarded the Nobel Prize for Literature, deals with this subject). In their 1926 published paper, Cole and Kuttner gave further experimental evidence to confirm the viral aetiology of this disease, named *cytomegalia infantum* [12]. These researchers induced the production of cells containing nuclear inclusion bodies, as they are seen in herpes simplex and related conditions, by injecting material from infected submaxillary glands of guinea pigs, first filtered through a Berkefeld N filter, which was impermeable to bacteria, into the brain of anesthetized guinea pigs, less than 1 month old. They concluded therefore that the infective agent belongs to the group of filterable viruses [12].

1.3 From 1930 to 1960

Sidney Faber and S. Burt Wolbach [13] from the Department of Pathology, Harvard Medical School, and the Pathology Laboratory of the Children's Hospital, Boston, summarized in 1932 in their paper the reports on intranuclear and cytoplasmic inclusions published until that. They noted that the distribution of the inclusions in the various organs of the reported instances was as follows:

Kidneys	11 cases
Parotids	10
Lungs	8
Liver	8
Pancreas	2
Thyroid	3
Intestine	1
Sublingual gland	1
Epididymis	1

In a table they included, they listed not only the authors and the location of the inclusion bodies but the year of publication, the pathological diagnosis and the interpretation of the findings. Chronologically, beginning 1904 with Jesionek and Kiolemenoglou, 'gregarines', 'amebae or sporozoa', 'coccidian', 'embryonic epithelial cells', 'endameba mortinatalium', 'peculiar epithelial degeneration', 'abnormal cytomorphosis "cytomegalia"', 'cellular degeneration', 'filterable virus' (Von Glahn and Pappenheimer), again 'protozoa' (Walz 1926) and, last but not least, 'undecided' (Wagner 1930) were listed under the heading 'Interpretation'. Faber and Wolbach themselves removed the submaxillary glands in a series of 183 postmortem examinations of infants and found intranuclear and cytoplasmic inclusion bodies in 22 cases (12%). This was the first indication that the infection by cytomegalovirus is highly frequent. In their summary they concluded that '. . .clinical and pathological studies of the series reported reveal no association with any distinctive feature or group of symptoms or disease changes. . .there are no distinctive clinical or pathological features which would permit its recognition on the wards or in the pathology laboratory'. This heterogeneous symptomatic, where almost every organ can be involved, and the pathology can vary from mild to almost life-threatening, is still a problem in diagnosis of cytomegalovirus disease [13].

By 1932, 25 cases of a rare lethal congenital infection characterized by petechiae, hepatosplenomegaly and intracerebral calcification had been described [14]. All of them had cells with typical intranuclear inclusions. The next two decades were dominated by the Great Depression and the Second World War. Mankind had other problems than cytomegalia in neonates and toddlers. The next step forward in the research of cytomegalia was done in the 1950s. This decade was coined by the Cold War, McCarthy, Marilyn Monroe and Elvis Presley. Concerning cytomegalia John P. Wyatt and his colleagues [15] formed for this disease in 1950 the term 'generalized cytomegalic inclusion disease' (CID). Since uniform sites of involvement were cells of the renal tubulus, they suggested that the disease might be diagnosed during life by searching for cells with inclusions in urinary sediments. Following this clue, Fetterman [16] made a cytologic preparation from 0.5 ml of urine obtained from a 3-day-old premature infant admitted to the Children's Hospital in Pittsburgh with jaundice, purpura, hepatosplenomegaly and intracerebral calcifications. He found several enormously hypertrophied cells with large intranuclear inclusions [16]. This was the first time diagnosis of cytomegalia could be done intravitum. The patient died at 4 days of age, and typical inclusions were found in the brain, pituitary, thyroid, lungs, liver and pancreas, in addition to the kidney, confirming the intravitum diagnosis of CID. W.H. Minder [17] reported in 1953 the results of electron microscope observations of pancreatic cells of a premature infant, who died 14 days after birth of CID, showing virus-like particles with a diameter of 199 nm in the nuclei and cytoplasm of infected cells. Although this was perhaps the first time the virus was seen, electron microscopy is hardly used for routine diagnostic, least of all in the 1950s of the last century. So, the technique of Fetterman, crude though it was, was better than no diagnostic technique at all. It was used with varying degrees of success for a number of years until the causative agent of the human disease was finally isolated [18].

The next milestone in the investigation of cytomegalovirus was the establishment of routinely growth of human cells in culture. The research on cytomegalovirus gained a great benefit from the work on poliovirus. John F. Enders, Frederick C. Robbins and Thomas H. Weller received the Nobel Prize in 1954 for this achievement. One year later, in 1955, Margaret Gladys Smith isolated from the submaxillary salivary gland of a 7-month-old infant dying of adrenal cortical carcinoma a virus which grew only in human but not in mouse cell culture. The paper describing this finding was rejected because she was also working with the mouse salivary gland virus and the editor thought her human agent might have been a mouse contaminant [14]. It is now known that cytomegalovirus is species specific and Margaret G. Smith was right and the editor was wrong.

Such misjudgements could occur nowadays as well; young scientists reading these words should learn from Margaret G. Smith not to lose courage but believe in their own work. It was only in 1956 when she re-isolated the virus and isolated the same virus from the kidney of a 1-month-old infant dying of generalized CID that her paper was accepted [19]. The changes she observed in the human fibroblast culture 4–7 days after oculation consisted of a few small, round or oval foci containing enlarged cells that were refractile, in contrast to normal fibroblasts. The lesions increased slowly in number and size. The centres of the lesions degenerated thereafter, leaving masses of dense, refractile granules. In fixed and stained preparations, large intranuclear inclusions were observed. Their shape usually corresponded closely to that of a nucleus. A clear, distinct zone separated the inclusion from nuclear membrane. Thus, the cytopathic changes closely resembled those seen in infected human tissues of patients with CID [7].

At the same time, Wallace P. Rowe and his co-workers in Bethesda studying the new group of adenoviruses by culturing adenoidal tissue observed an unusual type of cytopathology in the culture of adenoids from three children having tonsillectomy.

The cells in several tube cultures of each adenoid had spontaneous degeneration, characteristic of adenovirus infection, within 22 to 51 days. In one culture of each set, however, focal areas typical of a CMV infection developed after 34, 64 and 71 days of cultivation, respectively. The cytopathic changes resembled those observed by Smith. The isolated virus strain is still used as the AD169 (abbreviated from 'adenoid degeneration agent') laboratory strain of CMV [20, 21]. Contemporaneously in Boston Thomas H. Weller attempted to isolate *Toxoplasma gondii* in cell cultures. This protozoan causes a lethal congenital disease in neonates remarkably similar to CID clinically. From the liver biopsy of a 3-month-old infant with clinical signs suspected of toxoplasmosis, they wanted to isolate this infective agent. Nevertheless, the attempts to isolate *Toxoplasma* in roller cultures of human embryonic skin-muscle tissue were unsuccessful. Instead of this, the cultures showed foci of swollen cells after 12 days. Stained preparations showed cytopathology now associated with the salivary gland virus infection. The isolate is the now as Davis strain known cytomegalovirus strain [22].

Thomas H. Weller described this time in his paper published 1970 as follows [23]:

> The concurrent observation that poliomyelitis virus would grow in the skin-muscle suspended-cell system prepared for the varicella experiments brought many visitors to our laboratory. Among those, in May 1951, was Dr. Margaret Smith, who wished to apply the new methodology to the growth of the salivary gland viruses. ... by 1954 (she) had accomplished her objective of isolating and serially propagating human salivary gland virus from post-mortem materials. In contrast to the considered approach of Dr. Smith in St. Louis, the initial isolations of virus in Boston and in Bethesda were serendipitous. ... (In Boston) roller cultures of human embryonic skin-muscle tissue inoculated with ground liver tissue (of a 3-month-old infant with the "classical triad" of signs of congenital toxoplasmosis) did not yield Toxoplasma, but instead after 12 days showed foci of swollen cells. When stained, these foci revealed the intranuclear inclusions and cytopathology now associated with the cytomegaloviruses. ... (In Bethesda) in 1955, Rowe and co-workers were recovering a new group of viruses—the adenoviruses—by observing cytopathic changes in uninoculated cultures of human adenoidal tissue. Cultures of adenoids from 3 children developed unique changes that differed from those observed with the adenoviruses. ... The cytopathic changes resembled those we had described for varicella. Therefore, in May 1955, Rowe brought primary cultures of AD 169, set up on February 28, 1955, to Boston for study. ... As a result of Dr. Rowe's visit, strains of virus were exchanged, and the similarity of agents recovered in St. Louis, Boston, and Bethesda was established in advance of publication.

Although nowadays excellent collaboration in science exists too, this commendable cooperation should not be forgotten.

The propagation and isolation of the virus in cell cultures, showing the aetiology of CID, and the diagnostic tool Fetterman described, lead to a growing interest in this disease. Robert D. Mercer, Sarah Luse and Donald H. Guyton from Cleveland were the first who described a case of generalized cytomegalic inclusion disease in which the diagnosis was established during the life of the patient [24]. The patient died 5 weeks after admission. A. M. Margileth from the Department of Pediatrics, US Naval Hospital, Corona, California, was one of the first who described diagnosis and therapy of an infected newborn who survived. The examination of the microcephalic child at 14 months of age showed retardation in development. The patient was unable to sit alone, and moderate spasticity of the left hand and arm was noted. The treatment suggested was the administration of cortisone and gamma globulin [25]. Margileth concluded optimistically that '...we now have methods of diagnosing and treating cytomegalic inclusion disease of the newborn'. He did not know that he and other scientists working in this field did see at that time only the tip of the iceberg. And he did also not know that half a century later, there is still discussion of screening, diagnosis and therapy of congenital CMV infection.

The increasing interest in cytomegalic inclusion disease is also reflected by the amount of papers listed in the scientific database. From the 1940s to 1950s, the number of reports dealing with this disease rose from 2 articles from 1940 to 1950 to 96 articles from 1950 to 1960.

1.4 From 1960 to the Present

A further increase of publications was seen in the 1960s. From 1961–1970 almost 320 papers with the subject 'congenital CMV' were published. During this exciting, turbulent and revolutionary time of great social and technological changes, great effort was made in the CMV research. The isolation of the virus in tissue culture led to the development of antigens for use in a variety of serologic test. First data on epidemiology were collected leading to the statement that nonfatal cytomegalic inclusion disease in the neonatal period is a more common entity than has heretofore been appreciated. It was also speculated that congenital cytomegalic inclusion disease is seen more frequently than congenital toxoplasmosis [26]. It was supposed that some 1% of newborn infants enter the world with an active infection as indicated by the presence of viruria [27]. Early in this 'epidemiologic period' of cytomegalovirus research, social impacts were suspected to influence the occurrence of primary infections in mothers. Stern reported on serological studies showing that primary CMV infection was twice as high in immigrant Asian women compared to native-born English women [28]. In a discussion between experts written down in 1972, Hanshaw and Dudgeon presumed that there might be 4000 or more cases of congenital CMV infection per year in the United Kingdom, compared to about 200 cases per year of congenital defects due to rubella and about 30–50 and 35 cases of toxoplasmosis and congenital syphilis, respectively [28]. Although the scientific community was aware of the importance of this disease, there was a shift of interest to the problem of cytomegalovirus as fatal complication after organ transplantation. In the context of transplantation (and HIV infection later on), more sophisticated diagnostic tools were developed, assays based on molecular biology allowed new insights and CMV-specific virostatic drugs were introduced to the clinicians. These changes led to a better understanding of congenital CMV too. Nevertheless, it seems that many clinicians working in the perinatal field still forget about congenital CMV. Wyatt astonished about this behaviour already in 1950 [15] supposed for this omission a failure to recognize its importance (since it is largely a 'pathologist' disease, or a 'paediatrician' disease, by all means a disease bothering the others). Second, precariousness in interpreting diagnostic test and helplessness in choosing the right therapeutic strategies might be the reasons for this ostrichlike policy. But now, more than 120 years after the first description of this disease, there is time to solve the problem affecting still thousands of children. There exist good preconditions to do so.

References

1. Ribbert H (1904) Ueber protzoenartige Zellen in der Niere eines syphilitischen Neugeborenen und in der Parotis von Kindern. Centralblatt für Allgemeine Pathologie und Pathologische Anatomie 15(23):945–948
2. Jesionek W, Kiolemenoglou C (1904) Ueber einen Befund von Protozoenartigen Gebilden in den Organen eines hereditär-luetischen Fötus. Münchener Medizinische Wochenschrift 51 (43):1905–1907
3. Witz J (1998) A reappraisal of the contribution of Friedrich Loeffler to the development of the modern concept of virus. Arch Virol 143(11):2261–2263
4. Rott R, Siddel S (1998) One hundred years of animal virology. J Gen Virol 79:2871–2874
5. Loeffler F, Frosch P (1898) Berichte der Kommission zur Erforschung der Maul- und Klauenseuche bei dem Institut für Infektionskrankheiten in Berlin. Centralblatt für Bakteriologie, Parasitenkunde und Infektionskrankheiten Abt. I 23:371–391
6. Beijerinck MW (1899) Ueber ein *contagium vivum fluidum* als Ursache der Fleckenkrankheit der Tabaksblätter. Centralblatt für Bacteriologie und Parasitenkunde Abt II 5:27–33
7. Riley HD (1997) History of the cytomegalovirus. South Med J 90(2):184–190
8. Goodpasture EW, Talbot FB (1921) Concerning the nature of "protozoan-like" cells in certain lesions of infancy. Am J Dis Child 21(5):415–425
9. Tyzzer EE (1906) the histology of the skin lesions in varicella. J Med Res 14(2):361–392
10. Lipschütz B (1921) Untersuchungen über die Aetiologie der Krankheiten der Herpes genitalis. Arch Dermatol Syph 136:428–482
11. Luger A, Lauda E (1921) Ein Beitrag zur Frage der Übertragbarkeit des Herpes zoster auf das Kaninchen. Med Microbiol Immunol 94(2–3):206–213
12. Cole R, Kuttner AG (1926) A filterable virus present in the submaxillary glands of guinea pigs. J Exp Med 44:855–873
13. Faber S, Wolbach SB (1932) Intranuclear and cytoplasmic inclusions ("protozoan-like bodies") in the salivary glands and other organs of infants. Am J Pathol 8(2):123–135
14. Ho M (2008) The history of cytomegalovirus and its diseases. Med Microbiol Immunol 197:65–73
15. Wyatt JP, Saxton J, Lee RS, Pinkerton H (1950) Generalized cytomegalic inclusion disease. J Pediatr 36:271–294
16. Fetterman GH (1952) A new laboratory aid in the clinical diagnosis of inclusion disease of infancy. Am J Clin Pathol 22:424–425
17. Minder WH (1953) Die Ätiologie der Cytomegalia Infantum. Schweiz Med Wochenschr 83:1180–1182
18. Dudgeon JA (1971) Cytomegalovirus infection. Arch Dis Child 46:581–583
19. Smith MG (1956) Propagation in tissue cultures of a cytopathogenic virus from human salivary gland virus (SGV) disease. Proc Soc Exp Biol Med 92:424–430
20. Rowe WP, Huebner RJ, Kilmore LK, Parrott RH, Ward TG (1953) Isolation of a cytopathogenic agent from human adenoids undergoing spontaneous degeneration in tissue culture. Proc Soc Exp Biol Med 84:570–573

21. Rowe WP, Hartley JW, Waterman S, Turner HC, Huebner RJ (1956) Cytopathogenic agent resembling human salivary gland virus recovered from tissue cultures of human adenoids. Proc Soc Exp Biol Med 92:418–424
22. Weller TH, Macauley JC, Craig JM, Wirth P (1957) Isolation of intranuclear inclusion producing agents from infants with illneses resembling cytomegalic inclusion disease. Proc Soc Exp Biol Med 94:4–12
23. Weller TH (1970) Cytomegaloviruses: the difficult years. J Infect Dis 122(6):532–539
24. Mercer RD, Luse S, Guyton DH (1953) Clinical diagnosis of generalized cytomegalic inclusion disease. Pediatrics 11:502–514
25. Margileth AM (1955) The diagnosis and treatment of generalized cytomegalic inclusion disease of the newborn. Pediatrics 15:270–370
26. Weller TH, Hanshaw JB (1962) Virologic and clinical observations on cytomegalic inclusion disease. N Engl J Med 266(24):1233–1244
27. Weller TH (1971) The cytomegaloviruses: ubiquitous agents with protean clinical manifestations (second of two parts). N Engl J Med 285(5):267–274
28. Hanshaw JB, Schultx FW, Melish MM, Dudgeon JA (1972) Congenital cytomegalovirus infection. Ciba Found Symp 10:23–43

Virus–Host Interaction for Defense and Transmission

2

Gabriele Halwachs-Baumann

Herpesviruses have coexisted with their host for millions of year, thus having enough time to become accustomed to each other. The common ancestor of the family *Herpesviridae* has been proposed as having existed 400 million years ago. A number of 44 genes have passed from this ancestor to its now-existing descendents, whereas the rest of the genes have accumulated at later stages and thus differ between the members of the family [1]. HCMV, which has the largest genome among the herpesviruses, has evolved as a branch in the phylogenetic tree about 90–100 million years ago [2], and it is hypothesized that the virus is co-speciated with its host. This long-lasting interaction of virus and human led to a complex network of action and reaction on both sides and might explain the remarkable degree of strain variation, as well as the numerous possibilities in virus and host protein interaction at all stages of virus replication. One factor of success of HCMV is this good adaption to its reservoir. Since the virus needs the human for its own replication, killing its host has no benefit for the virus. The much better way to survive over the time and spread all over the world is an untroubled "subtenancy." So, under normal circumstances, HCMV does no harm to its host, sleeping in the depth of the human body and waiting for an opportunity to spread to another individual.

2.1 The Virus

The classification of herpesviruses has been updated in 2005 and brought in a new taxonomic order ([3]; http://www.ictvonline.org). Morphologically, herpesviruses are distinct from all other viruses. A linear, double-stranded DNA genome of

G. Halwachs-Baumann (✉)
Department of Laboratory Medicine, Regional Hospital Steyr, Steyr, Austria
e-mail: gabriele.baumann@gespag.at

G. Halwachs-Baumann (ed.), *Congenital Cytomegalovirus Infection*,
https://doi.org/10.1007/978-3-319-98770-5_2

125–290 kbp is contained within a $T = 16$ icosahedral capsid, which is surrounded by a proteinaceous matrix dubbed the tegument and then by a lipid envelope containing membrane-associated proteins. Genetically, herpesviruses fall into three distinct groupings that are related only tenuously to each other. These groupings consist of viruses of mammals, birds, and reptiles, viruses of fish and frogs, and a single virus of bivalves [3]. In the order *Herpesvirales*, the *Cytomegalovirus* (also named as human herpesvirus 5) belongs to the family of *Herpesviridae* and the subfamily of *Betaherpesviridae*.

In the human cytomegalovirus, 71 viral and more than 70 host proteins were detected by mass spectrometric analyses of extracellular virions [4]. Besides these structural proteins, the massive CMV genome, which is approximately 50% larger than the genome of herpes simplex, encodes for an undefined number of nonstructural proteins (some authors mention that the CMV genome encodes over 230 proteins, thereunder ≈54 membrane proteins including 25 membrane glycoproteins [5]). The genome itself is organized into long and short unique regions, each flanked by inverted repeats [6, 7].

The replication of CMV is slow compared to other herpes viruses. CMV lytic gene expression, like that of the other herpes viruses, occurs in a temporally ordered cascade. In general terms, the virus entry process requires a receptor-binding step, an activation step, and a membrane fusion step [8]. For HCMV entry begins with virion attachment to the ubiquitously expressed heparin sulfate proteoglycans at the cell surface, followed by binding of the viral glycoproteins gB and gH/gL to one or more cellular receptor(s) including the integrin heterodimers α2ß1, α6ß1, and αvß3, the platelet-derived growth factor-α receptor (PDGFRα), and the epidermal growth factor receptor (EGFR) [9]. In the review of Falcao et al. [10], it is mentioned that the virus binds simultaneously and independently to EGFR (via gB) and αvß3 (via gH) to induce a coordinated cellular signaling which is necessary for viral entry. Virus–receptor interactions seem to be cell-type specific, explaining the broad cell tropism of the virus. EGFR, for example, seems to be a key receptor for viral entry and successful infection of CD34+ human progenitor cells (HPCs) [11], fibroblasts, and breast cancer cells, whereas the infection of dendritic cells is based on an interaction with the dendritic cell membrane protein DC-SIGN [12]. Entry into fibroblasts was described to be promoted also by PDGFRα [5] to which the gH/gL/gO complex binds [13]. Subsequent delivery of capsids into the cytoplasm requires fusion of the virus envelope with cellular membranes. This fusion is mediated either by the gH/gL/UL128–131A complex or the gH/gL/gO complex, whereupon gH/gL/UL128–131A mediates the entry into epithelial/endothelial cells and gH/gL/gO mediates entry into fibroblasts [5, 14]. Besides the difference in the necessary viral glycoprotein complex, the entry into fibroblasts occurs in a pH-independent manner via fusion at the cell surface. In contrast, entry into epithelial, endothelial, dendritic, and monocytic cells occurs through endocytosis followed by a pH-dependent fusion event [14, 15]. So the virus behaves like a thief using different picklocks to open different doors. Thereafter, the deenveloped capsids must be transported toward the nucleus. This trafficking must be active, since passive diffusion would take >200 years for 1 cm cytoplasm. The reason for this is the crowded cytoplasm which has a protein density of approximately 300 mg/ml, analogous to the viscosity of wet sand [16]. To overcome this problem, the virus acts like a pirate. The docking and boarding of the virus which are initiated by the coordinated interaction of viral glycoproteins (the core fusion machinery) with host receptors induce a cytoskeletal rearrangement inside the cell [16]. So the virus can walk along the microtubular highways by using molecular motor proteins (i.e., dynein). Using this cellular cargo transport via the microtubular highway, it takes in fibroblasts only a few hours for the virus to reach the perinuclear sites [17], recent investigations presuming only 30 min in fibroblasts and endothelial cells for this translocation of viral DNA [18]. In CD34+ HPCs the time after entry of HCMV DNA reaching the nuclei is said to be 8 h [18], whereas in monocytes it takes 3 days [18]. Once the virus has reached the nucleus, the lytic replication cycle starts. This lytic replication cycle can be divided into three steps:

1. Circularization, in which the termini of the linear double-stranded viral genome are fused
2. Replication, in which the circular DNA serves as template for DNA replication, which generates large DNA concatemers
3. Maturation, in which the concatemeric viral DNA is processed into unit-length genomes, which are packaged into capsids

The transcription of the DNA occurs in a cascade-like fashion, which is characterized by typical proteins. In the first phase of replication, immediate-early (IE) genes are transcribed in the absence of de novo synthesis of viral proteins. In CMV, these genes carry out key regulatory functions in permissive as well as in latent infection. These IE proteins, of which IE72 (IE1) and IE86 (IE2) are the major forms, are potent and promiscuous transactivators of gene expression. The expression of viral immediate-early genes commits the virus to the lytic replication program. They participate in multiple interactions with the host cell's transcription machinery and also interact with components of cell cycle and growth control pathways. Importantly, the expression of the IE proteins is also absolutely crucial for the correct expression of the early (E) and late (L) classes of CMV genes—without which infection is abortive. Proteins necessary for the replication of the viral DNA are expressed in the early phase. After DNA replication, late genes are expressed, most of which encode proteins necessary for the generation of progeny virions [19, 20]. In certain cell types, IE genes are silenced upon HCMV infection, resulting in a latent infection [21].

Looking on an electron microscopic image of a CMV-infected cell, one can see clusters of "mini donuts" (Fig. 2.1). These round particles with diameters of approximately 80–100 nm are nucleocapsids which are found in electron-dense trabeculae of the inclusion body inside the nucleus [22, 23]. These capsids can impress as a single ring, so-called B-capsid, which are immediate precursors of DNA-containing particles, so-called C-capsid, shown up as a double ring. The capsids are surrounded by the tegument, basically composed of the high molecular weight protein (HMWP, ~212 kDa; CMV UL48), the basic phosphoprotein (BPP, ~149 kDa or pp150; CMV

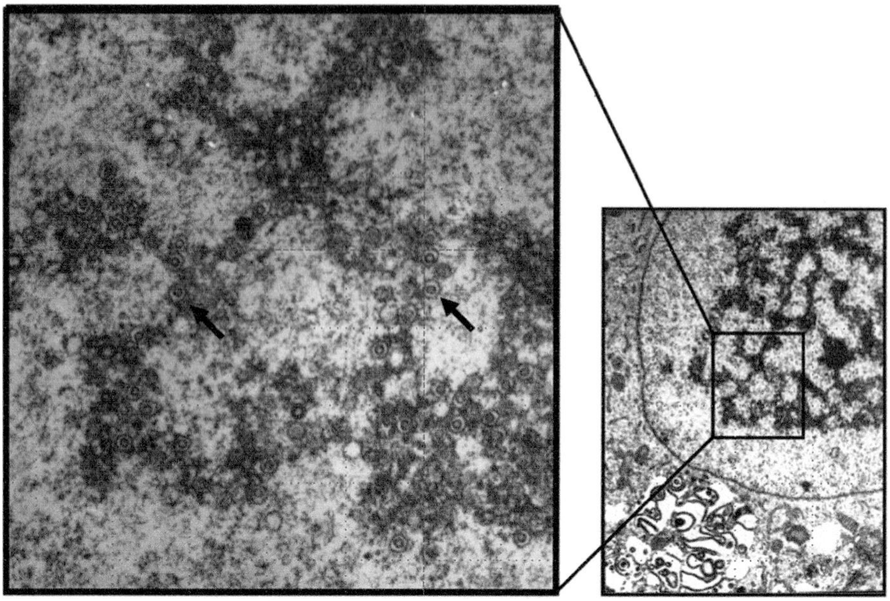

Fig. 2.1 Electron micrograph of a CMV-infected placenta cell (Trophoblast). The arrow is pointing at the virus

UL32), and the upper (72 kDa or pp71; CMV UL82) and the lower (69 kDa or pp65; CMV UL83) matrix proteins. With exception of the HMWP, each of the tegument proteins is phosphorylated and serves as a phosphate acceptor in vitro for the virion-associated protein kinase.

To leave the nucleus, the capsids get in touch with the inner nuclear membrane for budding. In the envelopment–deenvelopment model, this "primary" envelope is subsequently lost by fusion with the outer nuclear membrane resulting in the translocation of the nascent nucleocapsid into the cytosol (Fig. 2.2a). Besides this envelopment–deenvelopment model, the luminal modes exist, which proposes transit of the enveloped virion through the secretory pathway retaining its integrity [4].

After nuclear egress, the nucleocapsid has to acquire the full complement of tegument proteins and the final (secondary) envelope (Fig. 2.2c). This secondary envelopment is supposed to occur in so-called cytoplasmic "assembly compartments." The final viral envelope is acquired when the viral particles bud into Golgi apparatus-derived vesicles [21] (Fig. 2.3).

This secondary envelopment transforms B-capsids and C-capsids, respectively, into a noninfectious enveloped particle or into a mature virion surrounded by a double membrane (diameter 190–240 nm). The envelope of the virus contains at least eight different glycosylated proteins. Three of these originate from the CMV

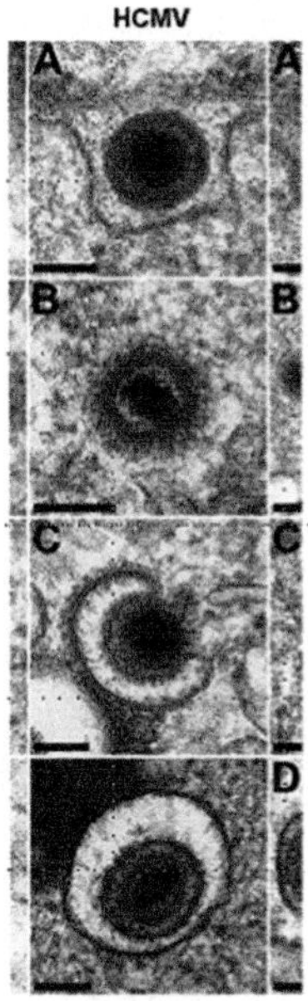

Fig. 2.2 Primary and secondary envelopment of HCMV. **(a)** Primary enveloped virions in the perinuclear space. **(b)** After translocation into the cytosol, capsids of HCMV are covered with a visible layer of the "inner" tegument. **(c)** Secondary envelopment and **(d)** presence of enveloped virions within a cellular vesicle during transport to the plasma membrane. Bar represents 100 nm. Reproduced from Mettenleiter et al. [1] with permission from Elsevier BV

gB gene (noncleaved gB, amino-cleavage fragments gB_N, and carboxyl-cleavage fragments gB_C). The fourth is the product of the gH gene. Further proteins are the gcIII, the gcII, and a 145 kDa glycoprotein referred to as the acidic glycoprotein, and the eighth envelope glycoprotein is called integral membrane protein (IMP) [23].

Furthermore, in addition to infectious virions, two other types of particles, noninfectious envelope particles (NIEPs) and dense bodies, are produced [21]. Dense bodies, i.e., effective virus particles, are enveloped aggregates of lower matrix protein (primarily pp65), lack capsids (and thus genomes), and vary in size from 200 to 1200 nm diameter [22]. In contrast to dense bodies, NIEPs are very similar to infectious virions, containing essentially identical proteins, but lack viral genomes [21].

At the last step of lytic infection, vesicles containing enveloped virions are transported to the plasma membrane, and subsequent virus is released by fusion of vesicle and plasma membrane (Fig. 2.3). This process needs interaction of the host microenvironment and viral tegument proteins, forming bridges between capsid-associated proteins and membrane-associated viral proteins [24]. Nevertheless, this process is not fully understood yet. Especially in polarized cells, it is a complex mechanism involving virus and host proteins, which has to be elucidated in detail.

Besides this described lytic virus replication, leading to clinical manifestations in immunocompromised or immunodefective hosts, the human cytomegalovirus is able to establish lifelong persistence following the initial, normally asymptomatic, infection in the immunocompetent human host. This latent infection is characterized at least in part by the carriage of the virus genome in the absence of detectable infectious virus. Importantly, this latent virus can routinely reactivate in vivo,

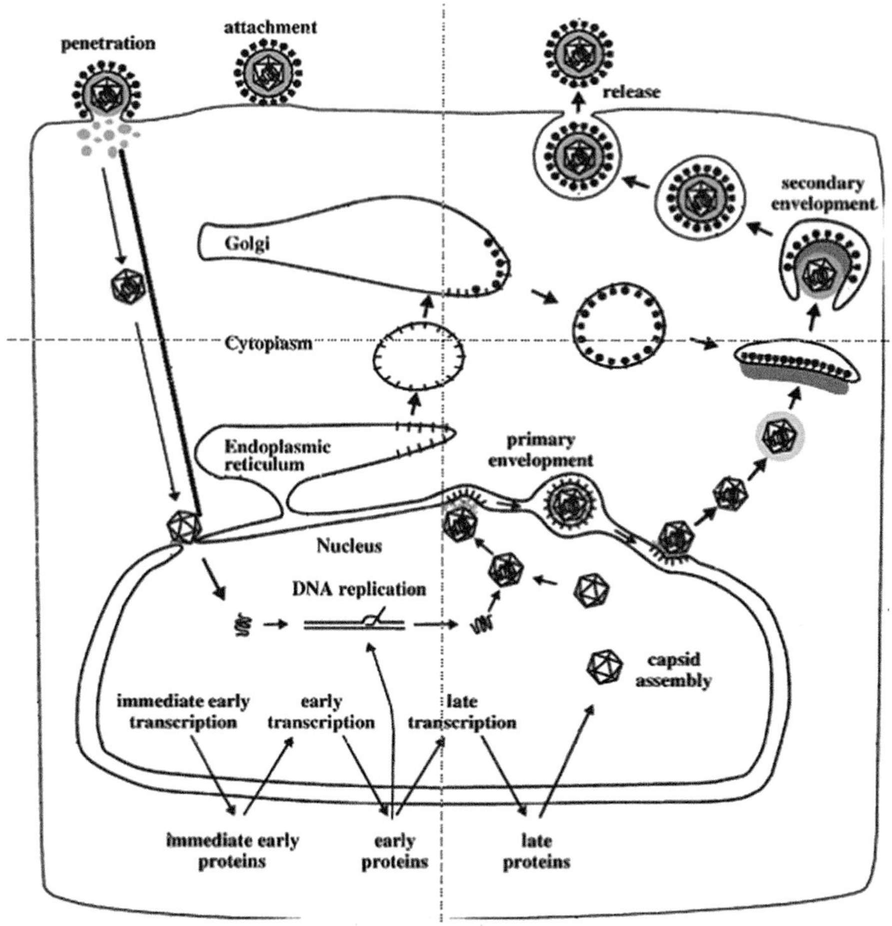

Fig. 2.3 Replication cycle of cytomegalovirus. Diagrammatic representation of the cytomegalovirus replication cycle, including virus entry and dissociation of tegument, transport of incoming capsids to the nuclear pore, and release of viral DNA into the nucleus where transcription occurs in a cascade-like fashion and DNA replication ensues

although these sporadic reactivation events, if they occur, are generally well controlled by the cell-mediated immunosurveillance. Important sites of latency in vivo are myeloid cells. It is now accepted that the suppression of viral lytic gene expression observed during latency in myeloid cells is a result of the inability of undifferentiated cell types to support robust viral immediate-early gene expression [25]. Recent experimental studies presume that also neuronal progenitor cells can act as sites of latency. The outcome of the infections seems to be dependent whether these cells are fetal or embryonic neuronal stem cells. These observations might be important for the understanding of the pathogenesis of neurological damage due to congenital CMV infection [26, 27]. Important for the establishment of HCMV latency is the silencing of the viral immediate-early proteins, which is controlled by a cellular intrinsic immune defense [28] via the regulation of the major immediate-early promoter (MIEP). The switch from latency to viral reactivation occurs when the MIEP is switched from a repressed to an active promoter state [26]. This seems to be promoted by cellular differentiation, which means that changes in the cellular environment are the stimulating reactivation event, which is assisted by inflammatory conditions. Besides latency (no productive infection), persistence (low-level productive infection) with little or no pathology or cell lysis can occur in different cell types [29]. The level of infection varies from cell type to cell type and is dependent on virus isolates. For instance, laboratory-adapted strains of CMV which have been routinely grown in primary human fibroblasts are unable to grow in myeloid, endothelial, or epithelial cells due to mutation or loss of one or more of the viral UL128–UL131A genes [25]. This UL128–UL131A locus is found to be highly conserved among field isolates. So the three encoded proteins seem to be all essential for growth of CMV in endothelial cells and virus transfer to leukocytes [30]. Besides differences between laboratory strains and field isolates, there exist also polymorphic sequences in coding and noncoding regions of the virus genome. This genetic variability among HCMV strains might explain differences in clinical manifestations of cytomegalovirus infections due to cell tropism of the virus and virulence. One of the most polymorphic gene among CMV clinical strains is the ORF UL73 encoding the immunogen envelope glycoprotein N (gN), a gC-II component implicated in virus attachment to the host cell and spread [31]. Since envelope glycoproteins like gN are targets for neutralizing antibodies, often produced with a strain-specific pattern and involved in virus entry and cell-to-cell virus spread, this heterogeneity of CMV is of interest in the context of congenital CMV infection.

2.2 The Host

2.2.1 Cell Types Involved in Replication and Distribution

All viruses, in contrast to other pathogens, can only live, i.e., replicate and thus survive, inside its host cell. For the cytomegalovirus this place of survival is tightly restricted to a species. That means human cytomegalovirus can only infect humans, mouse cytomegalovirus can only infect mice, etc. The focus of this book is only the human cytomegalovirus. If there are data reported from other species, this will be clearly mentioned.

The pathogenic effect in the individual host and the epidemiologic spread within a collective of hosts are inevitably linked to the spectrum of susceptible cell types. Although human cytomegalovirus is of pathologic relevance only for human beings, once the virus has entered its host, it can spread to virtually any tissue due to its broad range of target cell types (Fig. 2.4). This heterogeneity of susceptible cells explains the differences and diversity of clinical findings in CMV-infected persons (see above). The best-known cell type for CMV propagation is the fibroblast. Skin

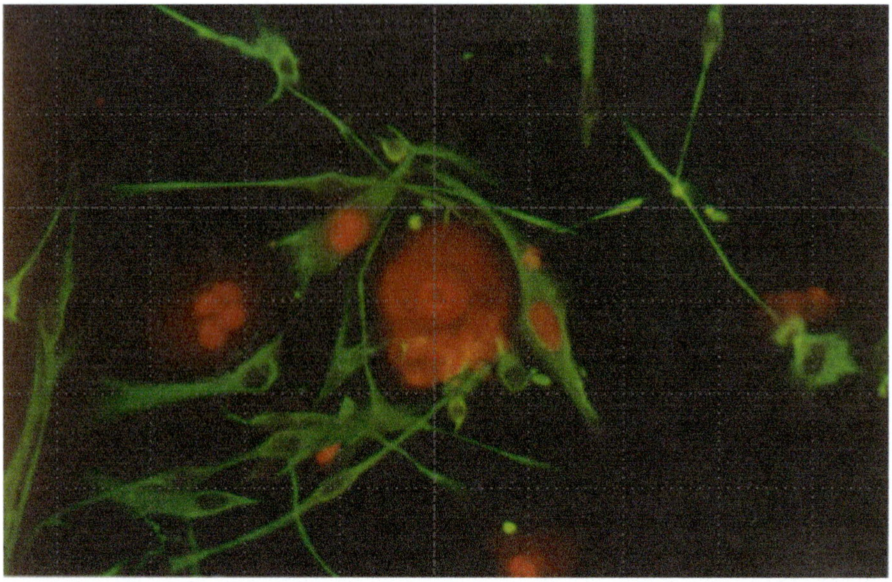

Fig. 2.4 Human trophoblast (red) infected with CMV, surrounded by CMV-infected fibroblasts (green)

fibroblasts and lung fibroblast were used in the first roller tube trials for the isolation and proliferation of clinical isolates in cell cultures. These strains are still used for experimental purpose and are now known as laboratory strains AD169 and Towne (see Chap. 1). In vitro cultured fibroblasts are still used to generate and release high titers of virus. This long-term culture of laboratory strains leads to the deletion of open reading frames within the UL128–131 regions, thus leading to a strong reduction of endothelial cell tropism, epithelial cell tropism, dendritic cell tropism, and virus transfer rate to granulocytes [32]. This phenomenon of interstrain differences in CMV cell tropism occurs as a cell culture artifact but leads to significant understanding of virus entry and virus spread in vivo. The fibroblast as reservoir of progeny virus is of particular impact not only as standard cell culture system for propagation of CMV. They are also among the major targets of CMV in vivo. Efficient replication in such an ubiquitous cell type opens the possibility for CMV to replicate in virtually every organ [32]. This explains the findings in bodies of neonates with fatal congenital inclusion disease [33]. Mesenchymal cells, which include also fibroblasts, were identified as target cells for CMV infection, and 39% (lung)—41% (pancreas) of infected cells seen in the involved organ belonged to this cell type. Compared to other cells (endothelial cells, epithelial cells, granulocytes, smooth muscle cells, etc.), mesenchymal cells (fibroblasts) were shown to be the predominant target cell of the CMV infection [33]. Recent studies have shown that also neuronal progenitor cells are susceptible for HCMV [27, 34].

To reach this site of high-titer viral progeny production and release, the virus has to cross the epithelial barrier which lines all external body surfaces. As it was shown for fibroblasts, epithelial cells are targets for CMV too [35]. The role of epithelial cells in CMV infection is that of a portal, where the virus can enter but also leave the host. As epithelial cells are polarized, i.e., divided into distinct apical and basolateral domains, susceptibility of these domains for CMV seems to be of importance. In the body, the apical surface faces the lumen of the organ and is separated by tight cell–cell junctions from the basolateral surface, which contacts adjacent cells or the underlying basement membrane. In polarized retinal pigment epithelial cells, tests of CMV infectivity showed that the apical membrane was 20- to 30-fold more susceptible to infection than the basolateral membrane [36]. In contrast to these observations in intestinal polarized epithelial cells, the virus enters predominantly through the basolateral surface [37]. Both directions of epithelial transit are necessary for CMV to survive efficiently in its preferred host cohort—the human being. In contrast to fibroblast, into which CMV enters by plasma membrane fusion, analysis of wild-type CMV strains shows that the virus enters epithelial (and endothelial) cells by endocytosis followed by low-pH-dependent fusion with endosomal membranes [38]. As abovementioned, this entry depends on the existence of genes UL128–131 (genes to the right, i.e., UL133–150 might also contribute to infection of epithelial and endothelial cells). These genes encode three small proteins with signal sequences that bind the CMV glycoprotein gH/gL. This gH/gL/UL128–131 complex, which is distinct from the gH/gL complexes containing the CMV glycoprotein gO, functions to mediate entry into epithelial and endothelial cells [39]. These differences in virus infection of fibroblasts and epithelial/endothelial cells are important for the understanding of defense mechanisms of the immune system, since UL128-, UL130-, and UL131-specific antibodies block infection of epithelial and endothelial cells but do not block infection of fibroblasts [40]. Moreover antibodies specific to gH block infection of fibroblasts [41].

After passing the epithelial barrier, the virus is able to infect (besides fibroblasts) organ-specific cells. The site of primary entry of the virus into the body can be the respiratory tract (host–host transmission of the virus via saliva or by hand–mouth inoculation), the gastrointestinal tract (host–host transmission of the virus via breast milk), or the urogenital tract (host–host transmission of the virus via sperm and cervical fluid). Keeping that in mind has important impact on prevention of CMV infection in mothers by increasing their awareness for hygienic actions. After a local passing of the epithelial barrier and a replication at the primary infection site, virus can pass the vessel wall by infecting vascular smooth muscle cells and vascular endothelial cells. Results from CMV DNA quantification in different blood compartments indicate further virus spread by different ways [42–44].

1. Free virus is transported in the blood plasma throughout the body. Systemic and symptomatic infection depends on virus load and immunogenic capacity of the host [42].
2. Transport by blood cells either by monocytes/macrophages or by polymorphonuclear cells. In healthy seropositive individuals, it was shown that <1 in 10,000

peripheral blood mononuclear cells carry the CMV genome. Of all blood leukocytes, peripheral blood monocytes are the major site of carriage [29, 45].

Sinzger et al. [32] assumed a tempting scenario where monocytes rolling along the vascular endothelium take up infectious virus from productively infected endothelial cells at one site of the body, differentiate upon transmigration through an activated endothelial layer at a different site of the body, and release virus progeny into the corresponding organ after maturation into tissue macrophages. This hypothesis might reflect one possibility of virus spread during active primary infection. Monocytes play a role not only in virus spread during primary infection but also in the case of reactivation of CMV in seropositive individuals. As with all lymphoid and myeloid cells, monocytes arise from pluripotent, CD34+ stem cells present in bone marrow. These CD34+ stem cells differentiate along the myeloid lineage to monoblasts, then promonocytes, in the bone marrow and then enter the bloodstream, where they lose CD34 cell surface antigen and develop into monocytes. Interestingly, CMV DNA can also be detected in such CD34+ bone marrow progenitors [29], and this carriage of viral DNA is not associated with lytic infection but is a true latent infection [46]. The differentiation of these myeloid progenitor cells specifically to dendritic cells leads to reactivated viral lytic gene expression and to the production of infectious virus [46], leading as a consequence to an anew viremic episode. However, the mechanisms regulating its latency and reactivation are not yet understood completely (see above). In the context of reactivation, the key inflammatory mediator IL-6 is described to have multiple effects, ranging from increased IE gene expression, less abortive reactivation events, and more efficient reactivation of infectious progeny [26]. In this context it seems to be important to mention that the IL-6 effect on reactivation is manifest only for cells being capable of supporting lytic infection to HCMV [47], whereas other studies have shown that only cells capable of supporting lytic infection produce and release IL-6 in higher amounts [48]. All these considerations sound a little bit like a hen-and-egg problem. Future will show what was first.

In contrast to monocytes/macrophages, polymorphonuclear cells can take up virus particles and express viral immediate-early proteins but do not support the full replicative cycle [49]. Although these cells cannot produce viral progeny, they are still capable of transmitting the infection to other cell types. Isolation of CMV from polymorphonuclear cells of immunocompromised patients gives evidence to this [50]. Thus virus recovery from leukocytes is the expression of virus passively transported by leukocytes, in the absence of degradation or inactivation [51]. The transmission of virus from endothelial cells to polymorphonuclear cells is supposed to be due to attachment and partial localized fusion of cell membranes with subsequent transfer of engulfed (sub)viral particles [32, 50]. Once chosen as vehicle by the virus, polymorphonuclear cells can transmit the virus to uninfected endothelial cells at random by the same mechanism but in the opposite direction.

Replication time in various cell types differs greatly as shown by in vitro experiments. Whereas in fibroblast the whole replication cycle is completed within 48 h, in endothelial cells it takes 72 h [20], and in hepatocytes nuclear inclusions representing late-stage cytopathic effects are detected at day 3 after infection [52]. In term trophoblast weak expression of late CMV antigen can be seen 120 h after infection [20]. So virus replication compared to other virus is very slow (the full replication cycle of rhinovirus takes 8–13 h) [53]. Furthermore, the way of the virus throughout the body is hampered by the immune system of the host.

2.2.2 The Immune System: Strengths and Weakness

During the coevolution of viruses and their hosts, the latter have equipped themselves with an elaborate immune system to defend themselves from the invading viruses. Facing the destructive consequences of microbial infections, the human immune system has evolved two arms of host defense designed to discriminate foreign agents and mount appropriate effector responses: the innate and the adaptive immune systems.

2.2.2.1 The Innate Immune System

Differing primarily in their receptors and receptor specificities, the innate immune system functions as the early and immediate defense mechanism and recognizes a broad set of conserved and invariant properties of nonself agents, such as viruses, through a diverse set of germ-line-encoded pattern recognition receptors (PRRs) [54]. One class of PRRs is the toll-like receptors (TLRs), of which to date 12 members have been identified in humans [55].

As mentioned above, there is a common sequence of processes that serve as the foundation for all viral infection. First, the infecting virus must migrate to the primary site of infection. In the case of CMV, this host–host transmission can precede by contact of mucosal secretions containing infectious virus of one person with the respiratory, gastrointestinal, or genitourinary tract of another person. In this context the salivary gland seems to be one major site of CMV harborage [56–58], and it could be presumed as one predominant portal for virus entry. As it was shown for fibroblast, the secretion of inflammatory cytokines and type I interferons from the host cell is the first and immediate reaction of the innate defense, and it occurs at the earliest points in the virus entry process—the virus binding to one or more cellular receptors. This binding is supposed to support multiple receptor–ligand interactions between viral envelope glycoproteins and cellular surface receptors, thus activating the inflammatory cytokine response through outright sensing by TLR2 irrespective of events needed for a productive infection [55]. Although the same mechanisms were not shown for CMV infection of epithelial cells, Bahri et al. [59] showed an equal phenomenon when gingival epithelial cells were pulsed with *Candida famata* in vitro. The expression and release of inflammatory mediators like IL-1β, TNF-α, and type I interferons lead to the recruiting of immune cells to the site of infection and the activation of the complement cascade. The complement system, in turn, has the task to induce inflammatory mediators, to opsonize pathogens, and to lyse directly pathogens and infected cells.

Mainly type I interferons, the first line of defense of the innate immune system, play a major role in spread and regulation of persistence of CMV. This IFN-I family consists of a dozen IFN-α subtypes, IFN-β, IFN-ε, IFN-ω, and IFN-κ, which have different functional differences [60]. In the mouse model in a view hours after infection, an increase of IFN-α/β can be observed [61]. This promotes upregulation of MHC and cosignaling ligands on bystander antigen-presenting cells, which represents a highly conserved link between innate and adaptive immune system. Nevertheless, IFN-I signaling is also associated with immunosuppressive events that lead to viral persistence. Vice versa blockade of IFN-β alone initiates events that lead to accelerated clearance of virus [60]. These findings redefine the paradigm of IFN-I as an exclusive host-protective, antiviral cytokine during viral infection. The cytomegalovirus as counterpart of the human cell tries to evade this first line of defense by influencing the human immune system for its own benefit. Once inside the target host cell, CMV prepares the cell for productive replication through two mechanisms: modulation of proinflammatory IFN cytokine production and reprogramming of cellular machinery. Immediately following entry, the tegument protein pp65, stored between the virion and surrounding envelope in the mature viral particle, is released and translocates to the nucleus, reducing the level of nuclear factor kappa B (NF-κB) production and blocking interferon regulatory factor-3 (IRF-3) activation [54]. Modulation of the IFN response is compounded by the activity of IE1-p72, a gene product expressed early after infection, which leads to the block of transcription of IFN-responsive genes. Another strategy of CMV to subvert innate immunity is the suppression of type I IFN production during primary viral infection via a CMV IL-10 homologue, thus mimicking the anti-inflammatory agency of IL-10. This viral IL-10 homologue released from CMV-infected cells potently inhibits IFN-α secretion by TLR9-activated plasmacytoid dendritic cells [59], a cell type producing normally up to 1000-fold more IFN-α in response to viral infection than other cell types. Additionally CMV also dramatically alters cellular gene expression and cell cycle progression immediately following infection, allowing for productive replication; the cell cycle is dysregulated and kept in a mitosis-like state, permitting early viral gene expression and productive replication of viral progeny before apoptosis occurs [54].

The complement system, another weapon of the innate immune system, consists of more than 30 soluble plasma and body fluid proteins and a number of cell receptors and control proteins found in blood and tissue [62, 63]. The complement system can be activated by the classical, alternative, or lectin pathways. All three pathways converge at the point of C3 cleavage and then generate the membrane attack complex C5b-9, leading to cytolysis. The activation of the complement system is followed by deposition of the complement opsonins, C3b and C3bi, on the surface of various pathogens, among other viruses. Specific receptors for both C3b (CR1) and iC3b (CR3) exist on phagocytes and promote the phagocytosis of microbes coated with opsonins [62]. These complement receptors CR3 (CD11/CD18) and CR4 (CD11c/CD18) are downmodulated in CMV-infected monocyte-derived macrophages, thereby altering the adhesion/phagocytic capacity of these cells [64].

The next force of the host to combat the virus is the natural killer cell (NK cell) arm of the innate immune system. NK cells surveil the host environment and are able to discriminate normal cells from those under duress or infection by monitoring the differential surface expression of MHC molecules on cells through the killer-cell immunoglobulin-like receptors (KIRs). Once downregulation of MHC expression is detected, ligation of the natural cytotoxic receptors (NCR) to viral hemagglutinin or unidentified ligands results in NK cell-mediated cytotoxicity and lysis of the affected cell [54]. Thus, normal self-recognition acts to suppress killing by NK cells, whereas a suppression of MHC molecules activates the NK cell. To evade this attack of the NK brigade, CMV induces the production of a MHC I homologue (gpUL18) in infected cells. This viral MHC I homologue binds to the NK cell inhibitory receptor LIR1/ILT2 with 1000-fold higher affinity than HLA-1 molecules, thereby inhibiting LIR1+ NK cells. Nevertheless, NK cell forces consist not only of LIR1+ cells but also of LIR1− cells. And these cells are stimulated by targets expressing gpUL18 [65]. HLA-E, a nonclassical MHC I molecule, acts in a similar manner as classical MHC I molecules. Expression on the surface suppresses NK cell-mediated cytotoxicity via binding to the NK cell inhibitory receptor CD94/NKG2A. HLA-E is also a potential ligand for the NK cell-activating receptor CD94/NKG2C. This dual function of the HLA-E molecule seems to provoke a dual evasion strategy of the virus. On the one hand, the CMV US6 protein blocks the transport of HLA-E-binding peptides to the ER by inhibiting the transporter associated with antigen processing (TAP) and thus inhibits HLA-E cell surface expression. To counter this vulnerability, the CMV glycoprotein encoded by UL40 upregulates the cell surface expression of HLA-E independent of TAP [65].

NK cells not only get their information via MHC I molecules. Other ligands for NK receptor exist (e.g., MICA, MICB, ULBP1–4, RAET1G, etc.). These ligands are expressed on the cell surface in response to stress, and CMV immediate-early proteins (IE1 and IE2) are particularly potent activators of this expression. As compensation to this signaling, dangerous for the virus survival, CMV encodes the gpUL16 (and presumably gpUL142 and gpUL141), which prevents cell surface expression of the abovementioned NK receptor ligands. Notably, gpUL141 is described to be the most robust modulator of NK cells that has been tested in vitro, inhibiting a wide range of human NK cell populations [66]. The effect of gpUL141 consists of sequestering the adhesion molecules CD155 and CD112 intracellularly, which are ligands for the NK cell-activating receptors CD226 and CD96 [66].

Quite different to these described receptor–ligand interactions is the function of the UL83 that encodes CMV tegument protein (pp65). As this protein is neither secreted nor expressed on the infected cell surface, the mode of operation starts after lysis of an infected cell, leading to an extracellular exposure of pp65 to the NK cell complex NKp30-ζ. Binding to this complex results in a dissociation of the signaling ζ-chain from the recognition of NKp30 receptor, which renders in an inhibition of NK cell activation [54, 65].

NK cells as a potent battalion of the innate immune system are aligned by antigen-presenting cells (APCs), which are pivotal in inducing adaptive immune responses. The cross talk between NK cells and APCs is bidirectional, since on the one hand, NK cells can kill immature APCs or promote their maturation and, in turn, mature APCs can stimulate NK cell cytotoxicity and proliferation [66]. Professional antigen-presenting cells present the antigen internalized either by phagocytosis or endocytosis on their cell surface bound to MHC II to T cells. Members of these professional antigen-presenting cells are dendritic cells, the most potent antigen-presenting cells of the innate immune system; macrophages, deriving from the same precursors as dendritic cells; certain activated epithelial cells; and B cell, as members of the adaptive immune system efficiently presenting the antigen to which their antibody is directed. Although all dendritic cells (DCs) are believed to arise from leukocytes derived from the hematopoietic compartment, they are not represented by any single uniform population of cells: location, phenotype, and specific immune function identify particular DC subsets. Two major DC subsets have been identified based on the differential expression of CD11c: the CD11c+ myeloid DCs, which are precursors for Langerhans DC, interstitial DC, and blood CD, and the CD11c– plasmacytoid DC, main producers of type I IFN [67, 68]. In the context of CMV infection, the interaction of antigen-presenting cells and the virus is like a double-edged sword. Apart from the possibility that CMV uses infected antigen-presenting cells as vehicles to travel to different tissues, the interactions between these cells and CMV play a dual role in immunity. On one hand, DCs (and macrophages) are essential for inducing a CMV-specific immune response, owing to their potent antigen-presentation properties and their unique capacity to stimulate T cells. On the other hand, DCs (and macrophages) are themselves targets for CMV, and by blocking their differentiation and blunting their immunostimulatory ability, the virus can evade the host immune response [67].

Antigen presentation, a crucial requirement for successful immune responses, relies on the major histocompatibility complex (MHC), in humans also termed human leukocyte antigen (HLA). MHC molecules are expressed on the cell surface and present short peptides to surveilling immune cells. The constitutive expression of class I molecules is distinct from that of class II molecules. In general, class I molecules are present on virtually all nucleated cells, whereas class II molecules are normally expressed only on B lymphocytes, macrophages, dendritic cells, endothelial cells, and few other cell types [69]. Peptides in the context of MHC class I are predominantly presented to CD8+ T cells, whereas MHC class II-restricted peptides are recognized mainly by CD4+ T cells. On MHC class I molecules, peptides are generated primarily by proteasomal degradation of cytosolic proteins and consecutively transported into the endoplasmic reticulum (ER) by the transporter associated with antigen processing (TAP). MHC class II molecules are instead loaded in lysosomes, where they associate with peptides derived from endocytosed exogenous proteins or endogenous proteins that enter the lysosomal compartment.

In CMV six different viral genes have been described to interfere with MHC class I (and II) pathways [70]:

The tegument protein pp65 prevents processing of the viral immediate-early antigen-1 (IE1) for presentation.

The US2 and US11 genes downregulate MHC class I molecules by rapidly translocating them to the cytosol, where they become tagged for proteasomal degradation.

US3 retains MHC class I molecules and interferes with MHC class II.

US6 blocks TAP function, thereby preventing the loading of MHC class I molecules with peptides.

US10 is possibly involved in delaying intracellular MHC class I trafficking.

UL82, encoding pp71, has recently been suggested to possess additional functions besides its known role in viral replication, namely, to inhibit the transport of MHC class I between ER and *cis*-Golgi.

These mechanisms are operational in all infected cells expressing MHC classes I and II. DCs, to bypass these viral impediments, generated an additional antigen presentation, not restricted to MHC class II molecules and independent of self-infection. In these cells exogenous proteins can eventually gain access to MHC class I as well—a phenomenon termed cross-presentation. This pathway permits antigens that are normally loaded onto MHC class II molecules to enter MHC class I presentation pathway. Cross-presentation allows DCs to present viral antigens to CD8+ T cells without being infected themselves [67, 70]. In support of this hypothesis, TNF-α secreted by CMV-stimulated monocyte-derived DCs appears to induce apoptosis of infected fibroblasts, leading to efficient internalization of CMV-enriched apoptotic bodies by immature DCs and effective presentation of viral antigens to CD8+ T cells in vitro [53]. In vivo studies demonstrated a broad repertoire of CD8+ T cells with specificities against IE, E, and L proteins [71].

Since DCs are unique in their ability to induce primary immune responses by priming and activating naïve T cells, thus allowing the establishment of immunological memory, interference with DC function could promote viral spread by paralyzing the adaptive immune system. Therefore CMV evolved a more specific impairment of DC functions. The effects of CMV on dendritic cells depend on the state of maturation and on the DC subsets. Infection of immature DCs leads to increased cell death and altered chemokine receptor expression (CCR1 and CCR5 downregulation) leading to altered migration properties [70]. Moreover, the ability of DCs to migrate to the lymph nodes and presentation of antigen to T cells is blunted by the inhibition of the expression of T-cell costimulatory molecules such as CD80, CD83, CD86, as well as MHC classes I and II and reduction of CCR7 expression, resulting in a lack of antigen-specific stimulation of T cells and inhibition of Th1 and Th2 response [68, 70]. The effect of CMV on mature peripheral blood myeloid dendritic cells (CD11c+, CD123−) results, as observed in immature monocyte-derived DCs, in the reduction of CD80, CD86, and MHC class I and class II, whereas CCR7 expression is not effected. It also impairs T-cell proliferation in mixed lymphocyte reaction [68]. In most analyses, virus-induced soluble factors released from the infected mature monocyte-derived DCs appear to mediate these effects. HCMV infection of mature plasmacytoid DCs (CD11c−, CD123+) results in changes in phenotype that resemble partial differentiation. This includes CMV-mediated increases in expression of MHC class II as well as increases in expression of T-cell costimulatory molecules such as CD83 and increases in interleukin-6 and interferon-α. As for monocyte-derived DCs, these CMV-mediated effects blunt the ability of plasmacytoid DCs to present antigen to CD8+ T cells resulting in a lack of antigen-specific stimulation of the Th1 response. Nevertheless, these CMV-mediated effects on plasmacytoid DCs induce T-cell-dependent B-cell activation and stimulation [68], thus presumably contributing to the successful control of CMV in the overwhelming part of the population [70].

2.2.2.2 The Adaptive (Acquired) Immune System

As mentioned above there is a close interaction between innate and adaptive immune system. Communication between these two units occurs via soluble or membrane-associated messengers. The interruption of this transfer of information is the aim of the cytomegalovirus to evade the immune system. It is noteworthy that, despite these immune manipulative strategies, the inhibition of class I antigen presentation observed in cytomegalovirus-infected cells in vitro is not sufficient to prevent the induction of a broad repertoire of CD8+ cytotoxic T cells after natural infection. Even the concerted action of all immune subversive proteins during the early and late phase of viral infection is not enough to prevent immune recognition in the epitopes from cytomegalovirus-encoded proteins [72]. So in the immunocompetent host, the development of an adaptive immune system cannot be disabled by the cytomegalovirus. It is the most important and effective control mechanism of virus replication and hence in protection against disease.

The adaptive (or acquired or specific) immune system consists of lymphocytes and their secreted products, such as antibodies. Specific immune responses are classified into two types, based on the components of the immune system that mediate the response: (1) the humoral immunity, which is mediated by antibodies, responsible for specific recognition and elimination of antigens. These antibodies are produced by B lymphocytes and can be transferred to unimmunized individuals by cell-free portions of the blood, i.e., plasma or serum. (2) The cellular immunity, mediated by T lymphocytes. T lymphocytes are further subdivided into functionally distinct populations, i.e., helper T cells (CD4+) and cytotoxic T cells (CD8+). Resolution of acute infection in normal individuals is associated with persistent immunological reactivity for CMV-encoded protein antigens that is characterized by a high frequency of CMV-specific CD4+ and CD8+ T lymphocytes and stable levels of antiviral antibodies [73].

CD8+ T lymphocytes perform their appointed missions by sampling the protein content of a cell in the form of peptides of 8–11 residues bound to cell surface major histocompatibility complex (MHC) class I molecules, which are ubiquitously expressed. In contrast to MHC I is MHC II expression limited to antigen-presenting cells, B cells, and monocytes/macrophages, which present antigen to CD4+ T lymphocytes [74]. The CD8+ T lymphocytes enact their effector functions through lysis of infected or antigen-presenting cells and by localized delivery of cytokines to infected cells (particularly IFN-γ and TNF-α). If the host has previously encountered the virus, any freshly infected cell will present its viral antigens in the context of MHC class I to these already primed exterminators permitting more rapid clearance of virus-infected cells [75]. The predominant CD8+ T-lymphocyte response following CMV infection was initially proposed to be directed against a limited set of virus-encoded antigens. The three dominant targets of

CMV-specific CD8+ T lymphocytes were pp65 (UL83), pp150 (UL32), and IE72 (UL123) [76, 77]. Studies with ex vivo T-cell assays have allowed rapid profiling of T-cell responses, showing that CD8+ T lymphocytes react to a large panel of cytomegalovirus antigens expressed during different phases of replication [71, 72]. Although T-cell reactivity against pp65, pp50, IE1, glycoprotein B, and IE2 seems to form a substantial part of CMV-specific cytotoxic T-lymphocyte response, subdominant T-cell reactivity is directed toward pp28, pp150, pp71, and US proteins. About 40% of the total T-cell responses are constituted by pp65 and IE1; 60% is directed toward other antigens, even in the presence of known immune evasion functions encoded by US (unique short) 2, 3, 6, and 11 of CMV [72, 73]. These CMV evasion proteins cause the active destruction of newly synthesized MHC molecules. Within the US region, the glycoproteins US2 and US11 induce the rapid export of MHC class I heavy chains out of the ER into the cytosol, where they are destroyed by the proteasome. The US3 impairs the transport of MHC class I complexes from the ER to the cell surface. US6 prevents peptide loading of MHC class I molecules by binding to the luminal part of both TAP subunits [75]. The host is fighting back by cross-priming and cross-presentation (see above), thus overcoming the inhibitory actions of the CMV molecules [67, 70, 78].

Following primary infection large expansion of polyclonal, activated, and directly cytotoxic T cells is generated. Within a few weeks, the viral DNA load has been decreased, and many clones of responding T cells have contracted in size and disappeared. An oligoclonal population of cells is selected into memory. This clonal focusing occurs with the loss of lower-avidity T cells. Many cells re-express the CD45RA isoform and have permanently lost CD28 and CD27 expression. These clones initially selected into memory are very stable for years, probably decades and for life; however, the size of the T-cell population does increase with time (memory inflation) and in the very elderly can become very large. New T-cell clonotypes can also arise with time, thus broadening the clonotypic repertoire [79, 80]. For HCMV it was shown that T cells recognize at least 151 proteins in a donor population of 33 individuals of mixed MHC backgrounds. CD4 T cells recognize 125 proteins, CD8 T cells recognized 107 proteins, and 81 proteins are recognized by both [81]. So, the HCMV-specific T-cell response targets mostly proteins that have a low variability between different HCMV strains [82]. It is noteworthy that normal, HCMV-exposed individuals devote a median of 9.1% and 10.2% of their circulating CD4+ and CD8+ memory T-cell repertoires, respectively, to HCMV [79, 82].

For effective CD8+ T-cell response, the support provided by CD4+ helper T cells is essential. This cell type gets the information via MHC II-associated antigen presentation. In vitro and in vivo studies have shown that CD4+ cells precede the emergence of the CD8+ T-cell response 24 h up to several days [79, 83, 84]. Analysis of the CD4+ T-cell responses to CMV has lagged behind that of the CD8+ T-cell response. However, antigen-specific cells have been identified by intracellular cytokine production, showing that CD4+ T cells often respond to the same ORFs as CD8+ T cells (see above). Conventionally, CD4+ T-cell responses were thought to play an indirect part by providing T cell help in maintaining virus-specific CD8+ memory response and in generation of virus-specific antibody responses [71]. Another CD4+ T-cell subset are cytotoxic CD4+CD28− T cells, which have an Ag-primed phenotype and express the cytolytic molecules granzyme B and perforin. They produce IFN-γ in response to CMV-Ag but may also secrete TNF-α and IL-2 [79] and can execute CMV-specific cytotoxicity in a class II-restricted fashion [84]. These CD4+ cytotoxic T-lymphocyte responses were mainly directed toward highly conserved regions of the glycoprotein B and the glycoprotein H antigens [71].

CMV does not limit its subversive maneuvers to the MHC class I pathway. The virus interferes also with MHC class II expression in several ways, including degradation of MHC class II glycoproteins via gpUS2, interference with the CIITA/JAK/STAT pathway, inhibition of surface expression of the metalloproteases CD10 and CD13, and finally perhaps also via the IL-10 homologue UL111A [74, 85]. Mainly the production of the CMV IL-10 homologue, which may inhibit host production of cytokines including IFN-γ, TNF-α, IL-2, and granulocyte–monocyte colony-stimulating factor, could lead to a Th1/Th2 switch, since IL-10 is known to be inhibitory to the Th1 pathway [74]. This impairment of cellular immune response might contribute to the establishment of CMV latency in the host.

This change in Th1/Th2 activation might also affect the humoral immune response by B lymphocytes. Th1 cells, which secrete IL-2 and IFN-γ, stimulate the antibody response dominated by IgG2a. IgG2a opsonizes antigens for phagocytosis, since it activates complement and binds to FcγRI receptors on macrophages. Antibody isotypes triggered by Th2 cells, such as IgE and IgG4, neither activate complement nor bind to macrophage Fc receptors. Rather, these antibodies are involved in host defense mediated by non-phagocytic effector cells, such as mast cells and eosinophils [69]. The immune response of humans seems to be not uniform. Different individuals exhibit different immunodominant patterns of response to CMV, among which the Th1 type is the dominant response [86]. This Th1-dominated immune response can be induced by dense bodies and is independent of de novo viral protein synthesis, as it was shown in a mice model [87].

Whereas cytotoxic lymphocytes can eliminate infected cells, antibodies have the potential to both eliminate infected cells and prevent infectious virus from infecting a cell (neutralization). The importance of antibody response for diagnostic purpose led to significant insights in the kinetics of the antibody response against human cytomegalovirus-specific proteins and thus a better understanding of the function of the humoral immune mechanisms. These explorations showed that the synthesis and catabolism of CMV-specific antibodies is a highly dynamic and complex process, with major differences between primary and secondary infections. Apart from the well-known and ubiquitous existing different kinetic of IgM and IgG after primary and secondary infection, primary humoral immune response against CMV is characterized by a production of IgG directed against CMV-specific phosphoproteins and delayed synthesis of glycoprotein-specific antibodies. In secondary response, antibodies against phosphor- and glycoprotein-specific antigens develop simultaneously [88, 89]. Also the maturation of IgG after primary infection characterized by the avidity of the produced antibodies takes time. After a period of several weeks to several months within that the antibody production changes from low to high avidity, IgG avidity remains high. The difference between the avidity of IgG produced at the beginning of primary infection and produced during secondary infections can be used as diagnostic tool [90–92].

The broad spectrum of CMV proteins inducing a humoral immune response is further subclassified by varying immunogenicity. The most immunogenic antigens for the humoral immune response against CMV inducing high levels of antibodies are p52, pp65, pp150, and ppUL32 compared to those to the immediate-early antigens [89, 93]. Antibodies against these polypeptides are nonneutralizing in contrast to those against glycoproteins. High titers of glycoprotein-specific neutralizing antibodies are correlated with the clearing of CMV DNA from the blood and a better outcome [89]. Several envelope glycoproteins, including glycoprotein B (gB, UL55), glycoprotein H (gH, UL75), glycoprotein L (gL, UL115), glycoprotein M (gM, UL100), and glycoprotein N (gN, UL73), have been identified as targets for neutralizing antibodies [41, 94, 95]. Within this protein dependency of the neutralizing antibody response, there is an additional epitope dependency, best studied in gB. Four linear antibody-binding sites have been described for this protein [96]. Antigenic domain 1 (AD1) was the first antibody-binding site defined on gB, and antibodies specific for this domain bind to different substructures [97]. In part these gB-specific antibodies neutralize the virus in a complement-dependent manner [68].

Additionally to the antigen diversification, antibody-mediated neutralization of cytomegalovirus is strain specific [98] and differs in the capacity of blocking viral infections depending on the host cell type. In that context, antibodies that are epithelial entry specific like those directed against pUL131A, pUL130, and pUL128 appear to display a major CMV-neutralizing and dissemination-inhibiting activity [40, 99].

In the last years, the focus of interest in CMV-specific humoral immune response was the research of neutralizing antibodies, since all current vaccines that are clinically protective are dependent on neutralizing antibody responses [100]. In theory, antibodies, though being capable of neutralizing free virions, could fail to prevent cell-bound virus dissemination from the portal of entry to distant target tissues and also could fail in preventing cell-to-cell spread within tissues. Recently, it was shown in a mice model that polyclonal cytomegalovirus-specific antibodies not only prevent virus dissemination from the portal of entry but also inhibit focal virus spread within target tissues [101]. Alternative effector mechanisms of antibody-mediated antiviral control, such as antibody-dependent cellular cytotoxicity (ADCC), are likely to be suppressed in the model of the immunocompromised host. In an immunocompetent person, this mechanism, as well as other mechanisms, might contribute to the effectivity of CMV-specific humoral immune response.

As for other parts of the immune system, CMV has developed evasion mechanisms to escape from the humoral immune system during the millions of years coexisting with the human. Gardner and Tortorella [14] listed in their review the following immune evasion mechanism:

1. Strain polymorphism: Superinfection by multiple viral strains leads to an increased diversity of strains within the host. Initial CMV infection elicits an antibody response that may not effectively neutralize infection by alternate strains. This variable threshold of neutralizing potency may be influenced by polymorphisms in a specific region that significantly limit the efficacy of the

existing humoral immune response. As mentioned above gB has five antigenic domains, AD1–AD5. Mainly in AD1 and AD2 amino acid, changes have been identified between clinical strains, which leads to different binding behavior of monoclonal antibodies [102]. Also in the domain, AD4 mutations can be found influencing the neutralization capacity of antibodies [103]. As for gB also for gH and gN, strain-specific variations have been described [104, 105]. Thus, polymorphism of various virus antigens may contribute to antibody evasion and facilitate superinfection of CMV-positive individuals. Furthermore, neutralization of CMV by antibodies to certain epitopes in gH or gH/gL is strain as well as cell type dependent [106].

2. Epitope competition: The induction of both neutralizing and nonneutralizing antibodies that compete for the same antigenic region could lead to protection of susceptible envelope protein regions from neutralizing antibodies. For gB as an example, immunogenic regions may serve in part as a decoy to elicit a nonneutralizing immune response, whereby critical entry factors are coated and virus binding and entering cells is possible furthermore [14].
3. Fc receptor-mediated endocytosis: This mechanism seems to be important for the transplacental transmission. This presumption is based on the observations of Maidji et al. [107] showing that syncytiotrophoblasts from the placentas of mothers with high neutralizing titers contain viral DNA-positive vesicles in which IgG and CMV gB are co-localized. Interestingly, HCMV expresses at least three different IgG Fc binding proteins, which allow the evading of immune responses mediated by host Fc receptors. These viral Fc receptors can participate in antibody bipolar bridging, thereby protecting virally infected cells from antibody- and complement-dependent neutralization, antibody-dependent cell-mediated cytotoxicity, and granulocyte attachment [108].
4. Glycan shielding: As it is known for HIV and influenza virus, glycosylation of surface proteins can protect the virus from antibody-mediated neutralization. For the HCMV envelope protein gN, which is highly glycosylated, it was shown that deletion of oligosaccharides from gN had a significant impact on the susceptibility to virus neutralization by antibodies. This effect was not only seen for antibodies directed against gN but also for a number of monoclonal antibodies that have been shown to be directed at different envelope proteins. An obvious explanation could be the shielding of a fraction of epitopes on gB and gH by the glycans of gN, thereby impeding antibody access to selected epitopes [109].
5. Cell-to-cell spread: Although it is widely accepted that cell-to-cell spread of cytomegalovirus exists, the complex mechanisms are yet poorly understood. It is generally thought that this process involves the directed release of mature virus particles into the space between adjacent cells with the subsequent adsorption and entry into a neighboring cell. For cells connected to each other with tight junctions, the exposure of spreading virus to the external environment is short, and thereby the virus is not readily susceptible to neutralizing antibodies [110]. The functioning of this evasion mechanism is supported by publications showing that neutralizing antibodies are unable to inhibit this viral cell-to-cell spread in certain cells [106, 111, 112].

2.2.3 The Placenta: A Barrier?

In every species studied, there is a strict quarantining mechanism between the mother and the conceptus. This nowadays self-evident statement was first postulated in 1794 by Hunter [113]. In 1953 the "immunological paradox" was postulated by the later Nobel Prize winner Peter B. Medawar. This hypothesis is based on the classical self/nonself model leading to elimination of an infectious agent or rejection of the allograft, which conceptualizes the fetus as a semi-allograft [114]. In 1984 Gambel et al. [115] described in his review experiments which demonstrated that the placenta serves as a specific immunoabsorbent barrier for antipaternal MHC class I antibodies and to maternal white blood cells while allowing red blood cells across. The special immunological situation of the maternal–fetal interface and recent hypothesis on this unique situation of mutual acceptance will be focused below. The realization of this continuous barrier between mother and fetus raised the necessity of transport mechanisms conquering this barrage. In a teleological sense, certain requirements had to be met in designing the maternal–fetal placental frontier [116]. The cellular membrane needed has to perform functions such as:

1. Transport of substances in both directions.
2. The regulation of osmotic gradients.
3. The maintenance of discretely different internal environments in the fetus and the gestating mother.
4. Maintenance and self-renewal.
5. The fashioning of its integral membrane proteins and other components in such a way that it would neither incite an effective cytotoxic immune response nor be susceptible to one, should an immune state exist in the parasitized host. The placental trophoblast, which is the dialysis membrane between the fetal and maternal circulations in hemochorial placentas, meets these requirements [116].

The human placenta itself is a fetomaternal organ, which differs from other organs in being formed by the interaction of both fetal and maternal tissues and being of limited life-span [113]. At term it is a local, disk-like thickening of the membranous sac that is formed by splitting of the membranes into two separate sheets, the chorionic plate (at the fetal side) and the basal plate (at the maternal side). These two plates confine the intervillous space, serving as cover and bottom. The intervillous space is perfused with maternal blood, which circulates directly around the trophoblastic surfaces of the placental villi. The villi are complex tree-like structures of the chorionic plate that project into the intervillous space. Inside the villi are fetal vessels that are connected to the fetal circulatory system via the chorionic plate and the umbilical cord. At the placental margin, the intervillous space is obliterated, so the chorionic plate and the basal plate fuse with each other and thus form the chorion laeve [117]. Nearly all maternofetal and fetomaternal exchange takes place in the placental villi. Despite differing functional specializations throughout placental development, all villi exhibit the same basic structure. The outer layer, separating the maternal blood from the villous interior, consists of trophoblasts. The trophoblast is composed of syncytiotrophoblast and cytotrophoblast. The syncytiotrophoblast consists of a continuous, uninterrupted, multinucleated layer without separating cell border. Between syncytiotrophoblast and its basement membrane are single or aggregated cytotrophoblastic cells, the Langhans cells, which are the stem cells of the syncytium, supporting the growth and regeneration of the latter. Two pathways give rise to the differentiated trophoblast cells that are found in floating and anchoring chorionic villi. In the pathway that gives rise to floating villi, cytotrophoblasts differentiate by fusing into multinucleated syncytiotrophoblasts. This trophoblast population is specially adapted for transporting a wide variety of substances to and from the embryo or fetus [118]. Cytotrophoblasts in the anchoring villi remain as single cells that aggregate into columns and invade the endometrium and the first third of the myometrium (interstitial invasion). They also breach portions of maternal arterioles that span these regions (endovascular invasion). By midgestation, invasive cytotrophoblasts have completely replaced the endothelial lining and much of the smooth muscle wall of these arteries, forming a hybrid vasculature composed of fetal and maternal cells [119]. During placental development, a molecular differentiation program is initiated that is required for normal pregnancy. Syncytiotrophoblasts and cytotrophoblast have a tremendous number of functions, making them the outstanding multitasking cells. Besides metabolism of steroid hormones (syncytiotrophoblast with prevailing smooth endoplasmic reticulum and syncytial lamellae covering Langhans cells), the complex, active maternofetal transfer of nutritions, including catabolism and resynthesis of proteins and lipids, synthesis of proteo- and peptide hormones (syncytiotrophoblast with prevailing rough endoplasmic reticulum), and diffusional transfer of gases and water, as well as facilitated transfer of glucose (vasculosyncytial membranes) belongs to duties of the syncytiotrophoblast layer [117]. Additionally Fcγ receptors (FcγR) are expressed on the syncytiotrophoblast as well as other cells of the placenta to provide active transfer of maternal IgG, NK cell activation, and transcriptional activation of cytokines [120]. These immunological activities of the placental cells will be discussed in detail below.

The trophoblastic basement membrane separates the trophoblast from the stromal core of the villi. On a minimum three cell layers and the basal membrane separate the intervillous space from the fetal blood. In the correct order, these are the syncytiotrophoblast layer, the cytotrophoblast, the basal membrane, and the endothelium from the fetal vessel [117].

The stroma is composed of varying numbers and types of connective tissue cells, connective tissue fibers, ground substance, and fetal vessels of various kind and caliber. The basic architecture of the villous stroma is constructed of fixed connective tissue cells that form a network. Mesenchymal cells, or undifferentiated stromal cells, are the prevailing cell type until the end of the second month. At the end of the second month, dramatic changes in stromal architecture and cellular composition take place. Within a few days, numerous small reticulum cells form that represent the prevailing cell type in the immature intermediate villi until the end of pregnancy. In stem villi and in smaller numbers in terminal villi and immature intermediate villi surrounding the larger vessels, fibroblasts can be found. Another cell type, which makes up nearly all of the cellular constituents of human villous stroma, is the myofibroblast. Furthermore, fetal tissue macrophages, the so-called Hofbauer cells, can be seen in the villi first on day 18 *post conceptionem* until gestation [117].

Besides the transport of nutrition and blood gases across the trophoblastic barrier, maternal immunoglobulins are other important macromolecules which have to pass from the maternal bloodstream to the fetal circulation. The immunoglobulins in the fetus consist almost totally of maternal IgG and are transferred across the placenta by means of a large number of different receptors. The distribution and function of these receptors differ on the various involved cell types. On syncytiotrophoblasts and on placental endothelial cells, the neonatal Fcγ receptor (FcRn) is expressed [121–124] and involved in the transfer of IgG. This FcRn is homologous to MHC class I molecules composed of an integral membrane glycoprotein with an apparent molecular weight of 40–45 kDa, the α-chain that is non-covalently associated with β2-microglobulin [124, 125]. The binding of IgG to the FcRn is pH dependent: at pH of 6.0, there is high affinity for IgG; at neutral pH, like it is in maternal blood, the affinity of the FcRn is 100-fold lower for IgG [122, 124]. IgG, present at high concentrations in the maternal blood (10–20 mg/ml), is internalized via fluid-phase endocytosis by the syncytiotrophoblast, followed by binding to FcRn in the acidic environment of endosomes [121, 124]. These coated vesicles protect IgG against a lysosomal proteolysis, thus allowing intact IgG to be released into the fetal circulation [123]. It was shown in placental endothelial cells that FcRn distinguishes between intact and modified IgG and controls their cellular traffic: native IgG is salvaged and released out of the cells, whereas modified IgG is retained and sorted to a degradative pathway [121]. Immunoglobulin (Ig) transport can be already seen in early embryos, at 3.5–5 weeks [126]. This transport leads to a continuous rise in the level of IgG (and IgA). At 17–22 weeks of gestation, fetal levels of IgG are only 5–10% of maternal levels. At term IgG levels exceed maternal levels by threefold [123, 127]. In parallel to the increase of fetal IgG levels, maternal levels of IgG and IgA decrease throughout pregnancy to a level of 60–70% of the initial concentration in early pregnancy [128]. From the IgG subclasses, IgG1 is the predominant immunoglobulin in the fetal circulation, followed by IgG4 and IgG3. IgG2 has a slow linear rise throughout pregnancy, but fetal IgG2 levels remain significantly below maternal concentrations [128]. In contrast to normal pregnancies, where mainly IgG passes through the placental barrier (to a lower extent, IgA is transported, no transport of IgM), in moderate inflammation, transport of IgG and IgA, and to a lesser degree IgM, increases. In cases with severe inflammation, transport of all types of Igs increases, with IgG showing the highest level [126].

Besides FcRn other Fc receptors (mainly FcγRI–III) are involved in the transfer of Igs and immune complexes. These receptors are found on fibroblasts and Hofbauer cells of the villous stroma which are involved in the binding and trapping of immune complexes [129]. On Hofbauer cells FcγR subtypes (I–III) are expressed; on endothelial cells mainly, FcγRII (and in some experiments FcγRIII) can be seen; and on trophoblast FcγRIII (besides FcRn) is the dominant Fc receptor on the surface [120]. The FcγRIIIa molecule on trophoblasts binds primarily immune complexes or antibody-coated particles in the maternal circulation and may associate with the transcription of lymphokines or the triggering of cell-mediated immunity [120, 129]. This receptor is also found on Hofbauer cells, just as FcγRIa and FcγRIIa. All three receptors mediate the endocytosis of immune complexes and would therefore enable Hofbauer cells to clear antibody–antigen complexes [129]. The same business seems to have the FcγRII on fetal vessel endothelium, i.e., clearing immune complexes. This trapping of immune complexes is efficient, because their concentrations in cord blood are below maternal levels, and there is little evidence for the transport of complexed antigens [129].

Continuing the idea of the placenta as a barrier and the trophoblast as the wall defending the unborn from every harmful influence, it can be said in the words of Moffett and Loke that we should consider the maternal immune response to be providing a nurturing balanced environment which curbs excessive or unsocial behavior by both placenta and mother leading to a state of peaceful coexistence between the two allogeneic tissues [130]. This unique immunological situation which arose during evolution seems to be supported by a so-called good inflammation, which is part of the "inflammation paradox" (in contrast to the "immunological paradox" of Medawar) postulated by Chavan et al. [114]. Since inflammation occurs as reaction after destruction of cells, irrespective of the source of destruction, and since implantation happens through destruction of maternal tissue, it is understandable that implantation of the human blastocyst activates the inflammation pathway [114]. Within the scope of these events, the decidua is populated by a large variety of leukocytes, accounting for >40% of the total cellar content. Unlike acute inflammation, implantation is not associated with neutrophil infiltration [114]. The major leukocyte population is represented by non-cytotoxic NK cells (>70% of decidual leukocytes) [131]. These decidual NK (dNK) cells, which are devoid of cytolytic activity, produce a large range of cytokines and chemokines and angiogenic factors, which play a major role in the recruitment and attraction of fetal trophoblasts. So dNKs promote vascular growth in the decidua through the production of vascular endothelial growth factor (VEGF), placental growth factor (PlGF), angiopoietin 1, angiopoietin 2, and TTGF-β1. The release of these factors depends on the engagement of NKp30- and NKp44-activating receptors by their specific ligands, which are present on the stromal decidual cells and extravillous trophoblast. Also the engagement of KIR2DL4, another NK cell receptor, by soluble HLA-G-specific ligand was shown to induce the production of proangiogenic cytokines. Migration of the extravillous cytotrophoblast into the decidua basalis is promoted by the release of interleukin-8 (IL-8) and interferon-inducible protein-10 (IP-10) chemokines which are also released by dNK. Such production of chemoattractants by dNK is due to the engagement of NKp30 and NKp44 by their specific ligands expressed by trophoblast and stromal decidual cells [132]. Besides this dNK cells have the ability of allorecognition, i.e., cross talk with the semi-allogeneic trophoblast in a way that induces tolerance of the conceptus. So, dNKs are crucial for the placental development and outcome of pregnancy. Besides this difference to "normal" inflammation, in implantation a different pattern of prostaglandins is produced. In contrast to "normal" inflammation, PGE_2 signaling is emphasized, and $PGF_{2\alpha}$ is reduced during eutherian implantation [114]. Because $PGF_{2\alpha}$ also induces contraction of myometrial smooth muscles during parturition, and luteolysis, suppression of $PGF_{2\alpha}$ is a key event in the recognition and acceptance of pregnancy [114]. Not all of the similarities and differences between inflammation and implantation are known yet, but the concept of the "inflammation paradox" seems to be a new way of reckoning the role of the maternal immune system during pregnancy, perhaps also in the context of congenital HCMV.

2.2.4 Cytomegalovirus–Placenta–Fetus: A Slippery Slope Between Defense and Transmission

As it was shown dramatically in those newborns infected intrauterinely with cytomegalovirus, the placenta is an imperfect immune barrier between mother and fetus. Despite nutrients and immunoglobulins, microorganisms like virus can cross the placenta. The route the virus takes across the placenta is yet not understood completely. Macroscopic investigations of placentas from mothers who gave birth to CMV-infected children showed grossly unremarkable findings; microscopically some chorionic villi exhibiting focal villous inflammation, necrosis with neutrophils, and nuclear debris were found. Plasmacytic infiltrates were found below the syncytial bordure either perivascular or in groups of 3–10 cells in the mesenchyme. Few of the affected villi contained definitive cytomegalic inclusion bodies [133–138]. Immunocytochemical studies demonstrated CMV immediate-early protein in endothelial cells, trophoblast cells, mainly cytotrophoblasts and cytotrophoblast progenitors, macrophages, and fibroblasts [139–141]. On the decidual site, invasive cytotrophoblasts, endothelial cells, macrophages, stromal decidual cells, and dendritic cells were shown to be infected with HCMV [142]. Also amniotic epithelial cells can be persistently infected with HCMV [143].

In vitro experiments with primary villous term and first-trimester trophoblasts have demonstrated the whole CMV replicative cycle in multinuclear syncytiotrophoblasts, but the infection requires high virus titers and proceeds slower than in fibroblasts [20, 144]. Infectious virus is released by trophoblasts and transmitted to adjacent uninfected fibroblast [20]. Interestingly the release of progeny virus from polarized trophoblasts is higher on the apical side, than on the basal side ($<1\%$). These findings suggest that very little CMV is released into the villous stroma where the virus could infect the fetus. An infection of the outer syncytiotrophoblast layer in the absence of collaborative events would thus be of little consequences. The trophoblast would act as a sink for the virus, retaining it until the trophoblast is sloughed off into maternal circulation through normal trophoblast turnover [145]. This hypothesis could be one explanation for the phenomenon that only in about 50% of primary CMV infection of the mother the unborn child is infected. Yet in every second in primary maternal CMV infection, the virus crosses the placenta. This takes about 3 weeks, as it was shown in explants of first-trimester human placenta, and the virus is passed from the trophoblasts to stromal fibroblasts and fetal endothelial capillary cells [146]. There seem to exist two distinct pathways of viral entry, i.e., fusion at the cell surface and endocytosis. Both mechanisms might lead to a higher probability of survival in solid tissues by potentially allowing immune evasion [142].

In the case of CMV infection of the placenta, the virus alters and modifies trophoblast cell functions. This alteration of the placental function can lead to miscarriage, stillbirth, and retardation of the fetal growth and brain. The alteration of normal transforming growth factor-β (TGF-β) production by trophoblasts might be one consequence of placental HCMV infection. Abnormal TGF-β1 disrupts the balance between the inhibition and stimulation of trophoblast cell differentiation and invasion, thus, resulting in poor pregnancy outcomes [147]. Furthermore, HCMV induces upregulation of the chemokine monocyte chemotactic protein-1/MCP-1 (CCL2) and TNF-α expression. This could lead to fetal injury, or even fetal demise, by either placental insufficiency due to shallow placentation or diminished function of the syncytiotrophoblasts, increased maternofetal virus transmission due to a disturbed syncytiotrophoblast barrier, adverse downstream effects on other proteins important for successful pregnancy, or loss of immune tolerance to the semi-allogeneic placenta [148].

This virus–trophoblast interaction depends on the gestational age, since the composition of the maternal–fetal barrier changes as pregnancy progresses. These stage-dependent differences in the effect of CMV infection on placental development and function were also shown morphologically [149]. Thus, in early pregnancy cytotrophoblast cells primarily form the maternal–fetal barrier, but later in gestation the continuous syncytiotrophoblast layer forms the major barrier between the maternal blood and the fetal capillaries [150]. As in other cell types and organs, the innate immune response is activated via toll-like receptors. This signaling through TLRs results in NF-κB activation and proinflammatory cytokine expression [151]. Proinflammatory cytokine release and the expression of adhesion molecules like ICAM-1 enhanced in CMV-infected syncytiotrophoblast lead to attracting and activation of decidual NK cells and monocytes [152–154], which leads to elimination of CMV-infected cells. This immune inflammatory reaction might also lead to disorders of the placenta (see above), shown also morphologically by an excessive accumulation of leukocytes in the intervillous/villous space, diffuse villitis, intervillitis, and extensive calcification of the villous plate [149].

In CMV infection virion-mediated activation of cells is triggered by the interaction of TLR2 and CD14 [155] with the viral surface proteins gB and gH [156]. In cells lacking either of these molecules (TLR2 and CD14), CMV was unable to activate the NF-κB pathway or trigger inflammatory cytokine production [151]. In placental trophoblasts the distribution of TLR2 and CD14 differs. Villous syncytiotrophoblasts facing the intervillous space strongly express TLR2 and use CD14 as a co-receptor for HCMV [157]. In contrast to syncytiotrophoblasts, cytotrophoblast expresses CD14 and TLR2 at much lower levels [157].

Binding of even ultraviolet-inactivated CMV to TLR2 and CD14 induces NF-κB activation and the release of TNF-α. This TNF-α release leads to apoptosis of infected syncytiotrophoblasts and neighboring uninfected cells, a host defense strategy designed to limit cell-to-cell spread of the invading pathogen. In the case of placental CMV infection, the removal of cytotrophoblasts leads to a damage of the placental trophoblast barrier [157–160]. Besides TNF-α, other proinflammatory cytokines, like IL-6 [48] and IL-8 [161], can be released by CMV-infected trophoblasts. Also amniotic epithelial cells infected with HCMV produce IFN-β, which could limit virus spread. Contrariwise in these cells, infection with HCMV upregulates the anti-apoptotic protein surviving and Bcl-x_L, whereby a host defense mechanism is affected, which should dispose damaged cells [143]. As for TNF-α, this cytokine release is observed in the absence of virus replication and results in cell death mainly of neighboring cells [162]. Interestingly IL-8 levels seem to be CMV strain dependent, since certain CMV strains induced higher levels of IL-8 in syncytiotrophoblasts than others [161]. It was observed by the same authors that IL-8 in turn enhances productive CMV expression in the placenta. It was also mentioned that IL-8 provided by coinfection agents or co-cultured macrophages [163] might have the same effect. This hypothesis could explain the observations of enhanced productive CMV infection of the placenta in the presence of coinfecting bacteria and virus [164–166].

The loss of trophoblastic cells at the maternofetal interface and the enhanced release of proinflammatory cytokines might either curtail the infection or lead to villitis, often seen in CMV-infected placentas and to an impaired function of the placenta [149]. As a result fetal loss, preterm labor, or intrauterine growth retardation can occur as consequence of placental CMV infection independently of fetal infection. Furthermore, the disruption of the trophoblast might act as a gate for CMV-infected maternal blood cells, leading to propagation of the virus in the placental stroma. In placental fibroblasts it was shown that CMV infection upregulates the cell surface expression of the tumor necrosis factor-related apoptosis-inducing ligand (TRAIL) via type I IFN through the NF-κB signaling pathway [167], a mechanism similar as in trophoblast, leading to apoptosis of infected cells, thus limiting virus spread. Interestingly in an ex vivo model of HCMV infection in human decidual tissues, maintained as multi-cell-type organ culture, it was shown that there exist differences in the innate immune response between the maternal, i.e., decidual side of the placenta, and the placental (fetal) villi. So IFN-γ induction was distinctive to the maternal decidua, whereas MxA and IP-10 were similarly induced in both tissues [168]. Generally there is an overall shift toward a proinflammatory environment starting with a robust tissue innate immune response within the whole-tissue decidual milieu. This shift toward a proinflammatory state was also observed in the amniotic fluid of congenital CMV-infected patients [169].

The activation of NF-κB not only induces the enhanced release of proinflammatory cytokines with the abovementioned consequences. This nuclear factor is also needed by the virus for the initiation of the gene cascade, as it was demonstrated in fibroblasts [170, 171]. The initial phase of NF-κB functions to "jump-start" viral gene expression immediately after infection, but also late CMV genes seem to contain NF-κB binding sites, since pp65 and gB expression can be blocked by inhibition of NF-κB activity [172]. So NF-κB activation by HCMV is a mixed blessing, leading to the rapid activation of the innate immune system and elimination of infected cells on the one hand, opening a possible gate for the virus to breach the trophoblast barrier and enhance virus replication on the other hand [55, 151, 173].

Besides the interaction of CMV gB and gH with TLR2 and CD14, other receptors for CMV entry on the surface of trophoblasts were described. Although discussed controversially [174–176] epidermal growth factor receptor (EGFR) with its co-receptor integrin β and αvβ3 was investigated on trophoblasts in the context of CMV infection. It was shown that the pattern of surface receptors differs between the various cell types of the maternal (uterine) and fetal (placental) site, which in turn seems to influence the pattern of CMV infection. Syncytiotrophoblasts expressing only EGFR and FcRn were abled for the uptake of IgG–virion complexes and for transcytosis. Floating villus trophoblasts expressing EGFR and αvβ3 showed focal infection. In the anchoring villus, in the proximal cell column, which expressed none of these receptors, no CMV infection at all was observed, whereas in the distal cell column expressing α1β1 and αV, virion binding was shown. On the maternal site, the interstitial/endovascular invasive cytotrophoblast expressing EGFR, αvβ3, and α1β1, productive CMV infection, and cell–cell virus spread was observed [177]. These findings indicate that virion interactions with cytotrophoblasts expressing receptors in the placenta:

1. Change as the cells differentiate
2. Correlate with spatially distinct sites of CMV replication in maternal and fetal compartments [177]

Despite the discussed role of EGFR and integrins as receptors for CMV, the major task of these molecules is the mediation of cell–cell and cell–matrix adhesion during migration. In the case of trophoblastic CMV infection, the differentiation and invasion capacities of these cells are impaired due to a downregulation of the key adhesion and immune molecules required for invasiveness [178]. Of note, CMV infection strongly and reproducibly altered trophoblast expression of mitotic cell cycle genes and strongly represses the expression of genes associated with trophoblast differentiation, particularly those associated with formation and stabilization of the extracellular matrix [179]. In early pregnancies the morphological counterpart to these molecular biological findings shown as pronounced dysmaturity of the villous structures was demonstrated [149]. This impairment of trophoblast migration and invasiveness is among others due to the interaction of the major immediate-early CMV promoter with the peroxisome proliferator-activated receptor gamma (PPARγ) of cytotrophoblasts, a nuclear receptor able to induce transcription of genes involved in lipogenesis and repression of genes involved in inflammatory processes [180]. Another explanation for the disturbance of cytotrophoblast function is the impairment of the extracellular matrix partly induced by the downregulation of matrix metalloproteinase (MMP) activity. MMPs are a family of degradative enzymes that remodel the extracellular matrix during many processes that include also the replacing of the walls of uterine spiral arterioles by invasive cytotrophoblast which populate the decidualized endometrium and the first third of the myometrium. This unusual process anchors the placenta to the uterus and supplies the fetus with maternal blood. The human cytotrophoblast produces the matrix metalloproteinase-9, absolutely required for cytotrophoblast degradation of and invasion through extracellular matrix. Cytokines and growth factors are involved in the tight regulation of normal and pathological events of placentation. IL-10, an anti-inflammatory cytokine, is inversely related to MMP-9 levels. It downregulates cytotrophoblast MMP-9 activity, thus inhibiting cytotrophoblast invasive capacity [181]. In differentiating-invading cytotrophoblasts and uterine microvascular endothelial cells, wild-type CMV strains, but not the laboratory strain AD169, downregulate MMP activity. This decrease of MMP activity and dysregulation of the cell–cell and cell–matrix interaction is induced via human IL-10 but also via cmvIL-10 [182]. In early pregnancy this inhibition of cytotrophoblast invasion may lead to impairment of placentation and restrict fetal growth, as well as other fetal and maternal pathologies associated with intrauterine CMV infection [183, 184]. Changes in the composition and function of the extracellular matrix of CMV-infected cells [179] in combination with the abovementioned changes in the immunological and inflammatory environment due to HCMV infection might have an impact to the transmission of HCMV to the fetus.

In the complex interaction between host and pathogen, the major histocompatibility complex molecules play a crucial role. In the placenta the situation is complicated, since the allogenic trophoblast cells are exposed directly to maternal immune effector cells, but the maternal immune system should not combat these cells. For many years, the absence of MHC-restricted rejection of the implanting trophoblast was attributed to the lack of MHC class I expression of these cells. It is now clear that trophoblast cells express both classical (HLA-C) and nonclassical (HLA-G and HLA-E) class I products [185, 186]. They contact with dNK cells by the inhibitory receptors, such as KIR2DL1, KIR2DL2 (for HLA-C), LIR-1 (for HLA-G), or CD94/NKG2A (for HLA-E), and help the fetal trophoblast cells escaping from being killed by the dNK [187].

HLA-G acts mainly to prevent NK cell cytotoxicity and induce tolerance, but also HLA-C, represented by allotype groups C1 and C2 and nonpolymorphic HLA-E, expressed at a low level by extravillous trophoblasts, is potent ligands for NK inhibitory receptors, i.e., CD94/NKG2A and specific killer-cell immunoglobulin-like receptors (KIRs) [188]. As mentioned above in the first trimester of pregnancy, 60–80% of decidual immune cells are NK cells. In contrast to peripheral NK cells, decidual NK cells (dNK) are $CD56^{bright}$, and do not express CD16 or CD3 but express high levels of the CD94/NKG2A inhibitory receptors. Furthermore, dNK expresses a repertoire of activating and inhibitory receptors (NKRs). One particularity of dNK cells is their ability to produce a large range of cytokines and chemokines and angiogenic factors, which plays a major role in the recruitment and attraction of fetal trophoblasts and in the early phases of decidual angiogenesis [131]. To deactivate the cytotoxic competence of dNK, the acquisition of HLA-G by dNK seems to be important. The cycle of HLA-G uptake by trogocytosis, internalization, degradation, and reacquisition by dNK induces a temporary knockout of cytotoxicity. Proinflammatory cytokine signals from HCMV infection seem to result in restoration of the cytolytic capacity of dNK by interrupting the HLA-G cycle [188, 189]. This functional and phenotypic change includes a downregulation of CD56 and an upregulation of CD16 expression on dNKs, changing the percentage of $CD56^{bright}$ to $CD56^{dim}$ from 95%:5% in normal decidua to 48%:40% in decidua infected with HCMV. Furthermore, an increased NKG2C+ expression on the surface of these cells is seen. On HCMV-infected decidual fibroblasts, an induction of NKp30-L and a decrease of NKp44-L and NKG2D-L expression [189] are seen, whereat "L" hallmarks the ligands for the appropriate surface receptor on the dNKs [132]. Interestingly, the upregulation of NKp44 on dNK and the downregulation of NKp44L on HCMV-infected decidual fibroblasts have a negative effect on dNK cytotoxic signals [132].

As mentioned above the interaction of NK cells with HLA-C leads to production of chemokines which contribute to trophoblast invasion [152]. In the case of a virus infection, normally the pathogen tries to escape detection by CD8+ cytotoxic T cells by interfering with the presentation of virus-derived peptides on MHC class I products at the surface of infected cells. In this case the downregulation would brand the virus-infected cell as MHC class I null cell and lead to the attack of NK cells [186]. In contrast to other MHC class I molecules, those MHC class I molecules expressed on the surface of trophoblasts (HLA-C, HLA-E, and HLA-G) are resistant to the effects of the CMV gene products US2 and US11, which normally downregulate class I surface expression by attaching to this molecule during synthesis. In consequence of this attachment, the newly synthesized MHC class I molecule is normally pushed backward in the endoplasmic reticulum and into cytosol. There it is deglycosylated, improperly folded, and degraded, not so in trophoblasts [186]. Importantly, trophoblasts HLA-G and HLA-C possess unique characteristics that allow their escape from CMV-associated MHC class I degradation. Trophoblast class I molecules could serve not only to block recognition by natural killer cells but also to guide virus-specific HLA-C- and possibly HLA-G-restricted cytotoxic T lymphocytes to their targets [185, 190, 191]. In the case of CMV, the virus tried to choose the lesser evil—NK cells dominate the leukocytes of deciduae by about 70%, whereas cytotoxic T cells are found only to a smaller extent [191]. Although at first glance the model of immune escape CMV evolved seems to be perfect, appearances are deceiving. Not the CMV gene products US2 and US11 downregulate trophoblast MHC class I molecules, but the CMV gene products US3 and US6 do so, namely, by two different mechanisms. CMV US3 physically associates with both trophoblast MHC class I species (HLA-G and HLA-C), retaining them in the endoplasmic reticulum. In contrast, CMV US6 inhibits peptide transport by transporter associated with antigen processing (TAP) and thus specifically the intracellular trafficking of class I molecules [192]. These differential regulatory mechanisms may create a balance of conditions optimal for the escape of viruses from CTL and for protection against NK cells [192]. But it might also create a condition where CMV-infected trophoblast is vulnerable to both CTL and NK cell attack.

In the last years, a number of papers were published dealing with the fine tuning of immune cells in placenta, which is necessary to find the way between assisting placentation and establishing immune tolerance to the conceptus on the one hand and defense against potential pathogens on the other hand. So, dNK cells respond to congenital HCMV infection by lowering the secretion of several soluble factors that are involved in trophoblast invasion, thereby limiting viral spreading and congenital infection [131]. It seems to be reasonable to slow down trophoblast invasion in the case of decidual infection, since decidual stromal cells (DSC) require an about tenfold less multiplicity of infection compared to extravillous trophoblasts and "separating" these two cell types increases the chance of destroying infected DSC before the virus can spread over to EVTs [193]. Furthermore, expression of KIR2DS1 by dNK increases the cytotoxic response of dNK to HLA-C2+ HCMV-infected maternal decidual stromal cells, preventing viral spread and placental pathology [193]. The importance of the matching between the HLA-C, HLA-E, and HLA-G genotype of mother and child and the KIRs expressed on dNKs was emphasized by the paper of Rovito et al. [194]. In their cohort, the maternal HLA-G del/del genotype was associated with a worse outcome of congenital HCMV infection, which might be explained by the immunosuppressive effect of this genotype. A higher percentage of symptomatic neonates were seen when there was a HLA-E*01012 mismatch (mm) and a HLA-C mm. Since HCMV peptides can be presented in the context of HLA-C and HLA-E, mismatches could lead to suboptimal viral clearance at the placenta. Furthermore, HLA-C non-inherited maternal antigens were associated with long-term impairments of the child, since the tolerance induced in the fetus toward these antigens may indirectly induce a suboptimal HCMV antiviral response throughout childhood.

Besides dNK cells T cells can be found in decidua. In early pregnancy these cells constitute 5–20% of total decidual lymphocytes. With gestational age this percentage increases. At full-term pregnancy 40–80% of decidual lymphocytes consist of T cells [188]; thereunder CD8+ T cells play the major role. These decidual CD8+ T cells seem to be antigen experienced and being highly differentiated cells. Interestingly the percentage of virus-specific CD8+ T cells in the decidua is significantly higher compared with peripheral blood. Although the role of these cells is not fully understood yet, the presence of these cells in the decidua seems to be important for the protection of the fetus from harmful infections by killing infected maternal cells in the placenta [188, 193, 195].

Taking together changes in the inflammatory response due to CMV infection of the placenta leads to a break of fetal–maternal tolerance and can lead to pregnancy complications by:

Impairment of trophoblast differentiation and invasiveness, leading to placental dysfunction, malnutrition of the fetus, preterm labor, or fetal loss
Enhanced expression of adhesion molecules and disturbance of the fragile cytokine milieu leading to villitis and placental dysfunction
Apoptosis of infected placental cells and uninfected surrounding cells, leading probably to disruption of the trophoblastic barrier, focal inflammation, and placental fibrosis/necrosis

So far the interaction between CMV, host immune system, and placental cells, as is the situation in primary CMV infection of the mother, was described. In secondary CMV infections of the mother besides cellular immunity, the presumably most valuable player—the humoral immune system—helps defending the virus. Epidemiologic investigations have shown that the presence of CMV-specific antibodies can reduce the transmission rate in case of active CMV infection of the mother from about 50% (primary infection) to about 1–2% (secondary infection). The same effect was seen in the case of passive immunization with CMV-specific immunoglobulins [196]. The mechanism of action of CMV-specific Ig is not completely understood. It probably includes:

1. Viral neutralization associated with high-avidity antibodies, thereby, for example, impeding the interaction of viral surface proteins (gB, gH, etc.) with their cell surface receptor
2. High levels of complement-fixing antibodies
3. Antibody-dependent cell-mediated cytotoxicity, reduced placental inflammation, and downregulation of cytokine-mediated cellular immune responses [197]

Since placental transfer of neutralizing antibodies is favored, compared to total CMV IgG antibodies, the beneficial effect of humoral immune response exists not only in the maternal but also in the developing fetal organism [198, 199]. Furthermore, in the presence of high-avidity CMV-specific IgG, viral replication in the placenta is reduced, thus reducing the probability of viral transfer to the fetus [151]. These data are supported by the observations of La Torre et al. [200], who observed that in women with primary infection, placental thickness was significantly increased, representing edema and inflammation induced by CMV. Administration of CMV hyperimmune globulin to women with primary infection was associated with significant reduction in placental thickness and improved placental health [200, 201]. Immunohistochemical staining of biopsy specimens from the deciduae and adjacent placenta showed differing pattern depending on the titers of

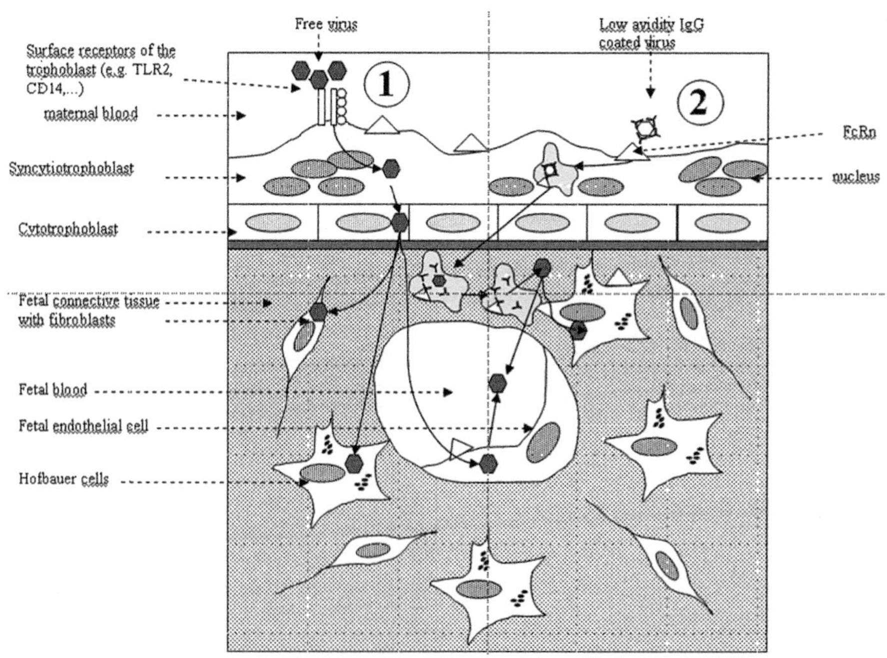

Fig. 2.5 Interaction between placenta and CMV-possible mechanisms. *1* CMV and surface receptor interaction (gB/gH with TLR2, CD14, etc.) and internalization of the virus. Virus replication and transmission to underlying cells (infection of placental fibroblasts, Hofbauer cells, endothelial cells). Release of the virus to the fetal circulation; *2* CMV coated with low-avidity IgG binds to the neonatal Fc receptor. Transcytosis of this complex. Release of the virus from its IgG coating in the acidic milieu of the vesicle. Free virus infecting placental cells

CMV-specific neutralizing antibodies. In specimen of women with low neutralizing antibody titers, cell islands in both compartments stained strongly for CMV replication proteins. In the decidua: glandular epithelial cells, cytotrophoblasts and resident decidual cells; in the adjacent portions of the placenta and floating villi: syncytiotrophoblast and cytotrophoblast progenitor cells were infected. Placental fibroblast and fetal capillaries in the villus core were infected too. In specimen of women with low to intermediate neutralizing titers, the number of cells with infected cell proteins was reduced in the deciduae, and occasional focal infection was found in the placenta. In samples from women with high neutralizing titers, only few infected cells were found in the decidua, and none were seen in the placenta. In the syncytiotrophoblast, villus core macrophages and dendritic cell gB-positive vesicles were found, but these cells were not infected [165, 184, 202].

Experiments gave evidence that the neonatal Fc receptor for maternal IgG expressed in early-gestation placentas might bind IgG–virion complexes from maternal blood in the intervillous space. These complexes might be transcytosed to underlying cytotrophoblasts [107]. Depending on the avidity of the neutralizing antibodies, either infection of these cells occurs in the case of low avidity, or CMV fails to replicate in the case of high avidity [107, 201]. As mentioned above immunoglobulins are internalized via fluid-phase endocytosis by the syncytiotrophoblast, followed by binding to FcRn in the acidic environment of endosomes. So one explanation for the discrepant action of high- and low-avidity neutralizing antibodies could be the phenomenon that virus–antibody complexes

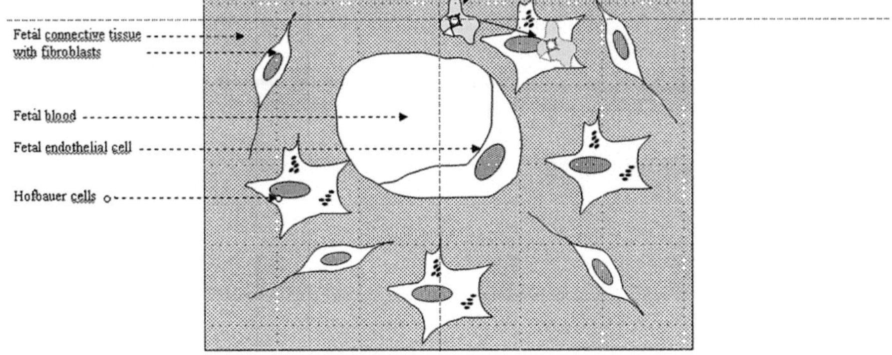

Fig. 2.6 Interaction between placenta and CMV-possible mechanisms. *3* CMV coated with neutralizing antibodies (anti-gB, anti-gH), thereby blocking the interaction of viral surface proteins with trophoblast surface receptors. No viral entry possible. *4* CMV coated with high-avidity IgG binds to the neonatal Fc receptor. Virus–immunoglobulin complex stays stable. Phagocytosis and degradation by villous macrophages

dissociate at low pH and the viral infectivity is restored by the use of acidic buffer (pH 4.8) [203]. So it can be hypothesized that the intact virus is released by low-avidity immunoglobulins more easily in the acidic milieu of the endosomes. High-avidity IgG binds tight to the virion even in an acidic milieu, and the virion–IgG complex is sorted to a degradative pathway, as it was shown for modified immunoglobulins [121], or phagocytosed by villous core macrophages [107].

Regarding the FcRn molecule as a possible gate for antibody-coated virions to cross the placental barrier, the downregulation of the neonatal Fc receptor by IFN-γ [204] could be interpreted as protection mechanism of the host.

Although the effect of CMV-specific immunoglobulins on the prevention of congenital CMV infection cannot be totally explained yet, it can be said that lowering the viral load in the maternal blood, preventing viral entry into the cell by blocking the various viral surface receptors, and forming robust antibody–virion complexes which are then phagocytosed and degraded seem to be three important characters of active produced as well as passive administered CMV-specific immunoglobulins.

Possible interactions between placenta and CMV for defense and transmission are illustrated in Figs. 2.5, 2.6, and 2.7.

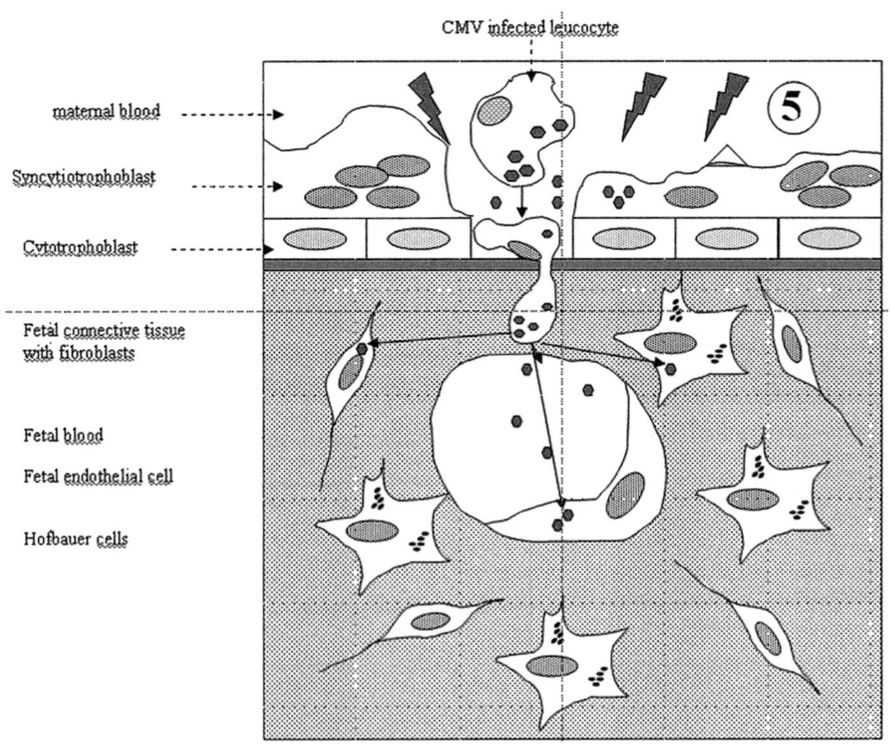

Fig. 2.7 Interaction between placenta and CMV-possible mechanisms. *5* Infection of trophoblasts with ensuing inflammation and apoptosis of infected cells. Leakage of the placental barrier, opening a gate for the passage of infected leukocytes and free virus

References

1. Davison AJ (2011) Human herpesvirus. In: Reed D. L., Currier R. W., Walton W. F., et al. The evolution of infectious agents in relation to sex in animals and humans: brief discussions of some individual organisms. Ann N Y Acad Sci 1230:74–107
2. Davison AJ (2002) Evolution of the herpesviruses. Vet Microbiol 86:69–88
3. Davison AJ, Eberle R, Ehlers B, Hayward GS, McGeoch DJ, Minson AC, Peooett PE, Roizman B, Studdert MJ, Thiry E (2009) The order Herpesvirales. Arch Virol 154:171–177
4. Mettenleiter TC, Klupp BG, Granzow H (2009) Herpesvirus assembly: an update. Virus Res 143:222–234
5. Vanarsdall AL, Johnson DC (2012) Human cytomegalovirus entry into cells. Curr Opin Virol 2(1):37–42
6. Ho M (1991) Cytomegalovirus: biology and infection, 2nd edn. Plenum Medical Book Company, New York
7. Plachter B, Sinzger C, Jahn G (1996) Cell types involved in replication and sitribution of human cytomegalovirus. Adv Virus Res 46:195–261
8. Sathiyamoorthy K, Chen J, Longnecker R, Jardetzky TS (2017) The COMPLEXity in herpesvirus entry. Curr Opin Virol 24:97–104
9. Miller MS, Hertel L (2009) Onset of human cytomegalovirus replication in fibroblasts requires the presence of an intact vimentin cytoskeleton. J Virol 83(14):7015–7028
10. Falcão ASC, da Costa Vasconcelos PF, Lobato da Silva DF, Viana Pinheiro JJ, Falcao LFM, Quaresma JAS (2017) Mechanisms of human cytomegalovirus infection with a focus on epidermal growth factor receptor interactions. Rev Med Virol 27(6):e1955. https://doi.org/10.1002/rmv.1955
11. Kim JH, Collins-McMillen D, Caposio P, Yurochko AD (2016) Viral binding-induced signalling drives a unique and extended intracellular trafficking pattern during infection of primary monocytes. Proc Natl Acad Sci U S A 113(31):8819–8824
12. Halary F, Amara A, Lortat-Jacob H et al (2002) Human cytomegalovirus binding to DC.SIGN is required for dendritic cell infection and target cell trans-infection. Immunity 17(5):653–664
13. Wu Y, Prager A, Boos S et al (2017) Human cytomegalovirus glycoprotein complex gH/gL/gO uses PDGFR-α as a key for entry. PLoS Pathog 13(4):e1006281
14. Gardner TJ, Tortorella D (2016) Virion glycoprotein-mediated immune evasion by human cytomegalovirus: a sticky virus makes a slick getaway. Microbiol Mol Biol Rev 80:663–677
15. Zhou M, Lanchy JM, Ryckman BJ (2015) Human cytomegalovirus gH/gL/gO promotes the fusion step of entry into all cell types, whereas gH/gL/UL128-131 broadens virus tropism through a distinct mechanism. J Virol 89(17):8999–9009
16. Lyman MG, Enquist L (2009) Herpesvirus interactions with the host cytockeleton. J Virol 83(5):2058–2066
17. Sampaio KL, Cavignac Y, Stierhof YD, Sinzger C (2005) Human cytomegalovirus labeled with green fluorescent protein for live analysis of intracellular particle movements. J Virol 79(5):2754–2767
18. Kim JH, Collins-McMillen D, Buehler JC, Goodrum FD, Yurochko AD (2017) Human cytomegalovirus requires epidermal growth factor receptor signaling to enter and initiate the early steps in the establishment of latency in CD34+ human progenitor cells. J Virol 91(5):e1206–e1216
19. Halwachs-Baumann G (2006) The congenital cytomegalovirus infection: virus-host interaction for defense and transmission. Curr Pharm Biotechnol 7(4):303–312
20. Halwachs-Baumann G, Wilders-Truschnig M, Desoye G, Hahn T, Kiesel L, Klingel G, Rieger P, Jahn G, Sinzger C (1998) Human trophoblast cells are permissive to the complete replicative cycle of human cytomegalovirus. J Virol 72(9):7598–7602
21. Kalejty RF (2008) Tegument proteins of human cytomegalovirus. Microbiol Mol Biol Rev 72(2):249–265

22. Grefte JMM, van der Giessen M, Blom N, The TH, van Son WJ (1995) Circulating cytomegalovirus-infected endothelial cells after renal transplantation: possible clue to pathophysiology? Transplant Proc 27(1):939–942
23. Gibson W (1991) Cytomegalovirus protein structure and function. In: Landini MP (ed) Progress in cytomegalovirus research. Elsevier Science Publishers, Amsterdam
24. Guo H, Shen S, Wang L, Deng H (2010) Role of tegument proteins in herpesvirus assembly and egress. Protein Cell 1(11):987–998
25. Sinclair J (2009) Chromatin structure regulates human cytomegalovirus gene expression during latency, reactivation and lytic infection. Biochim Biophys Acta. https://doi.org/10.1016/j.bbagrm.2009.08.001
26. Dupont L, Reeves MB (2017) Cytomegalovirus latency and reactivation: recent insights into an age old problem. Rev Med Virol 26(2):75–89
27. Pan X, Li XJ, Liu XJ et al (2013) Later passages of neural progenitor cells from neonatal brain are more permissive for human cytomegalovirus infection. J Virol 87(20):10968–10979
28. Saffert RT, Penkert RR, Kalejta RF (2010) Cellular and viral control over the initial events of human cytomegalovirus experimental latency in CD34+ cells. J Virol 84(11):5594–5604
29. Sinclair J, Sissons P (2006) Latency and reactivation of human cytomegalovirus. J Gen Virol 87:1763–1779
30. Baldanti F, Paolucci S, Campanini G, Sarasini A, Percivalle E, Revello MG, Gerna G (2006) Human cytomegalovirus UL131A, UL130 and UL128 genes are highly conserved among field isolates. Arch Virol 151:1225–1233
31. Pignatelli S, Dal Monte P (2009) Epidemiology of human cytomegalovirus strains through comparison of methodological approaches to explore gN variants. New Microbiol 32:1–10
32. Sinzger C, Digel M, Jahn G (2008) Cytomegalovirus cell tropism. Curr Top Microbiol Immunol 325:63–83
33. Bissinger AL, Sinzger C, Kaiserling E, Jahn G (2002) Human cytomegalovirus as a direct pathogen: correlation of multiorgan involvement and cell distribution with clinical and pathological findings in an case of congenital inclusion disease. J Med Virol 67:200–206
34. Luo MH, Schwartz PH, Fortunato EA (2008) Neonatal neural progenitor cells and their neuronal and glial cell derivatives are fully permissive for human cytomegalovirus infection. J Virol 82(20):9994–10007
35. Sinzger C, Greefte A, Plachter B, Gouw ASH, The TH, Jahn G (1995) Fibroblasts, epithelial cells, endothelial cells and smooth muscle cells are major targets of human cytomegalovirus infection in lung and gastrointestinal tissues. J Gen Virol 76:741–750
36. Tugizow S, Maidij E, Pereira L (1996) Role of apical and basolateral membranes in replication of human cytomegalovirus in polarized retinal pigment epithelial cells. J Gen Virol 77:61–74
37. Esclatine A, Lemullois M, Servin AL, Quero AM, GEniteau-Legendre M (2000) Human cytomegalovirus infects Caco-2 intestinal epithelial cells basolaterally regardless of the differentiation state. J Virol 74(1):513–517
38. Ryckman BJ, Jarvis MA, Drummond DD, Nelson JA, Johnson DC (2006) Human cytomegalovirus entry into epithelial and endothelial cells depends on genes UL128 to UL150 and occurs by endocytosis and low-pH fusion. J Virol 80(2):710–722
39. Ryckman BJ, Chase MC, Johnson DC (2008) HCMV gH/gL/UL128-131 interferes with virus entry into epithelial cells: evidence for cell type-specific receptors. Proc Natl Acad Sci U S A 105(37):14118–14123
40. Gerna G, Sarasini A, Patrone M, Percivalle E, Fiorina L, Campanini G, Gallina A, Baldanti F, Revello MG (2008) Human cytomegalovirus serum neutralizing antibodies block virus infection of endothelial/epithelial cells, but not fibroblast, early during primary infection. J Gen Virol 89:853–865
41. Urban M, Klein M, Britt WJ, Haßfurther E, Mach M (1996) Glycoprotein H of human cytomegalovirus is a major antigen for the neutralizing humoral immune response. J Gen Virol 77:1537–1547

42. Boeckh M, Boivin G (1998) Quantitation of cytomegalovirus: methodologic aspects and clinical applications. Clin Microbiol Rev 11(3):533–554
43. Ziyaeyan M, Sabahi F, Alborzi A, Ramzi M, Mahboudi F, Pourabbas B, Kadivar M (2008) Quantification of human cytomegalovirus DNA by a new capture hybrid polymerase cahin reaction enzyme-linked immunosorbent assay in plasma and peripheral blood mononuclear cells of bone marrow transplant recipients. Exp Clin Transplant 6(4):294–300
44. Preiser W, Brink NS, Ayliffe U, Peggs KS, Mackinnon S, Tedder RS, Garson JA (2003) Development and clinical application of a fully controlled quantitative PCR assay for cell-free cytomegalovirus in human plasma. J Clin Virol 26:49–59
45. Hassan-Walker AF, Mattes FM, Griffiths PD, Emera VC (2001) Quantity of cytomegalovirus DNA in different leukocyte populations during active infection in vivo and the presence of gB and UL18 transcripts. J Med Virol 64:283–289
46. Sinclair J (2008) Human cytomegalovirus: latency and reactivation in the myeloid lineage. J Clin Virol 41:180–185
47. Reeves MB, Compton T (2011) Inhibition of inflammatory interleukin-6 activity via extracellular signal-regulated kionase-mitogen-activated protein kinase signaling antagonizes human cytomegalovirus reactivation from dendritic cells. J Virol 85(23):12750–12758
48. Halwachs-Baumann G, Weihrauch G, Gruber HJ, Desoye G, Sinzger C (2006) hCMV induced IL-6 release in trophoblast and trophoblastlike cells. J Clin Virol 37(2):91–97
49. Grefte JMM, van der Gun TF, Schmolke S, van der Giessen M, van Son WJ, Plachter B, Jahn G, The TH (1992) The lower matrix protein pp65 is the principal viral antigen present in peripheral blood leukocytes during an active cytomegalovirus infection. J Gen Virol 73:2923–2932
50. Gerna G, Percivalle E, Baldanti F, Sozzani S, Lanzarini P, GEnini E, Lilleri D, Revello MG (2000) Human cytomegalovirus replicates abortively in polymorphonuclear leukocytes after transfer from infected endothelial cells via transient microfusion events. J Virol 74 (12):5629–5638
51. Gerna G, Baldanti F, Revello G (2004) Pathogenesis of human cytomegalovirus infection and cellular targets. Hum Immunol 65:381–386
52. Sinzger C, Bissinger AL, Viebahn R, Oettle H, Radke C, Schmidt CA, Jahn G (1999) Hepatocytes are permissive for human cytomegalovirus infection in human liver cell culture and in vivo. J Infect Dis 180:976–986
53. Rollinger JM, Schmidtke M (2009) The human rhinovirus: huma-pathological impact, mechanisms of antirhinoviral agents, and strategies for their discovery. Med Res Rev. https://doi.org/10.1002/med
54. Kim WM, Sigalov B (2008) Viral pathogenesis, modulation of immune receptor signalling and treatment. Adv Exp Med Biol 640:325–349
55. Juckem LK, Boehme KW, Feire AL, Compton T (2008) Differential initiation of innate immune responses induced by human cytomegalovirus entry into fibroblast cells. J Immunol 180:4965–4977
56. Campell AE, Cavanaugh VJ, Slater JS (2008) The salivary glands as a privileged site of cytomegalovirus immune evasion and persistence. Med Microbiol Immunol 197:205–213
57. Smith MG (1954) Propagation of salivary gland virus of the mouse in tissue cultures. Proc Soc Exp Biol Med 86:435–440
58. Smith MG (1956) Propagation in tissue cultures of a cytopathogenic virus from human salivary gland virus (SGV) disease. Proc Soc Exp Biol Med 92:424–430
59. Bahri R, Saidane-Mosbahi D, Rouabhia M (2009) *Candida famata* modulates toll-like receptor, ß-defensin, and proinflammatory cytokine expression by normal human epithelial cells. J Cell Physiol 222:209–218
60. Ng CT, Sullivan BM, Teijaro JR et al (2015) Blockade of interferon beta, but not interferon alpha, signaling controls persistent viral infection. Cell Host Microbe 17:653–661
61. Loewendorf A, Benedict CA (2010) Modulation of host innate and adaptive immune defenses by cytomegalovirus: timing is everything. J Intern Med 267(5):483–501

62. Rus H, Cudrici C, Niculescu F (2005) The role of the complement system in innate immunity. Immunol Res 33(2):103–112
63. Miller-Kittrel M, Sparer TE (2009) Feeling manipulated: cytomegalovirus immune manipulation. Virol J 6:4. https://doi.org/10.1186/1743-422X-6-4
64. Gafa V, Manches O, Pastor a, Drouet E, Ambroise-Thomas P, Grillot R, Aldebert D (2005) Human cytomegalovirus dorwnregulates complement receptors (CR3, CR4) and decreases phagocytosis by macrophages. J Med Virol 76:361–366
65. Wilkinson GWG, Tomasec P, Stanton RJ et al (2008) Modulation of natural killer cells by human cytomegalovirus. J Clin Virol 41:206–212
66. Rossini G, Cerboni C, Santoni A et al (2012) Interplay between human cytomegalovirus and intrinsic/innate host responses: a complex bidirectional relationship. Mediators Inflamm 2012:607276
67. Varani S, Frascaroli G, Landini MP, Söderberg-Naucler C (2009) Human cytomegalovirus targets different subsets of antigen-presenting cells with pathological consequences for host immunity: implications for immunosuppression, chronic inflammation and autoimmunity. Rev Med Virol 19:131–145
68. Sinclair J (2008) Manipulation of dendritic cell function by human cytomegalovirus. Expert Rev Mol Med 10:e35. https://doi.org/10.1017/S1462399408000872
69. Abbas AK, Lichtman AH, Pillai S (2007) Cellular and molecular immunology, 6th edn. Elsevier, Philadelphia, PA
70. Rölle A, Olweus J (2009) Dendritic cells in cytomegalovirus infection: viral evasion and host countermeasures. APMIS 117:413–426
71. Martin H, Mandron M, Davriche C (2008) Interplay between human cytomegalovirus and dendritic cells in T cell activation. Med Microbiol Immunol 197:179–184
72. Gandhi MK, Khanna R (2004) Human cytomegalovirus: clinical aspects, immune regulation, and emerging treatments. Lancet Infect Dis 4:725–738
73. Britt W (2008) Manifestations of human cytomegalovirus infection: proposed mechanisms of acute and chronic disease. Curr Top Microbiol Immunol 325:417–470
74. Froberg MK (2004) CMV escapes! Ann Clin Lab Sci 34:123–130
75. Basta S, Bennink JR (2003) A survival game of hide and seek: cytomegaloviruses and MHC class I antigen presentation pathways. Viral Immunol 16:231–242
76. La Rosa C, Wang Z, Lacey SF et al (2005) Characterization of host immunity to cytomegalovirus pp150 (UL32). Hum Immunol 66(2):116–126
77. Gibson L, Piccinini G, Lilleri D et al (2004) Human cytomegalovirus protiens pp65 and immediate early protein 1 are common targets for CD8+ T cell responses in children with congenital or postnatal human cytomegalovirus infection. J Immunol 172(4):2256–2264
78. Mandron M, Martin H, Bonjean B, Lulé J, Tartour E, Davrinche C (2008) Dendritic cell-induced apoptosis of human cytomegalovirus-infected fibroblasts promotes cross-presentation of pp65 to CD8+ T cells. J Gen Virol 89:78–86
79. Waller ECP, Day E, Sissons JGP, Wills MR (2008) Dynamics of T cell memory inhuman cytomegalovirus infection. Med Microbiol Immunol 197:83–96
80. van Leeuwen EMM, de Bree GJ, ten Berge IJM, van Lier RAW (2006) Human virus-specific CD8+ T cells: diversity specialists. Immunol Rev 211:225–235
81. Terrazzini N, Kern F (2014) Cell-mediated immunity to human CMV infection: a brief overview. F1000Prime Rep 6:28. https://doi.org/10.12703/P6-28
82. Sylwester AW, Mitchell BL, Edgar JB et al (2005) Broadly targeted human cytomegalovirus-specific CD4+ and CD8+ T cells dominate the momory compartments of exposed subjects. J Exp Med 202(5):673–685
83. Gerna G, Percivalle E, Lilleri D, Lozza L, Fornara C, Hahn G, Baldanti F, Revello MG (2005) Dendritic-cell infection by human cytomegalovirus is restricted to strains carrying functional UL 131-128 genes and mediates efficient viral antigen presentation to CD8+ T cells. J Gen Virol 86:275–284

84. van de Berg PJEJ, van Stijn A, ten Berge IJM, van Lier RAW (2008) A fingerprint left by cytomegalovirus infection in the human T cell compartment. J Clin Virol 41:213–217
85. Loenen WAM, Bruggeman CA, Wiertz EJHJ (2001) Immune evasion by human cytomegalovirus: lessons in immunology and cell biology. Semin Immunol 13:41–49
86. Zhu J, Shearer GM, Marincola FM, Norman JE, Rott D, Zou J-P, Epstein SE (2001) Discordant cellular and humoral immune responses to cytomegalovirus infection in healthy blood donors: existence of a Th1-type dominant response. Int Immunol 13:785–790
87. Pepperl S, Münster J, Mach M, Harris JR, Plachter B (2000) Dense bodies of human cytomegalovirus induce both humoral and cellular immune responses in the absence of viral gene expression. J Virol 74:6132–6146
88. Schoppel K, Kropff B, Schmidt C, Vornhagen R, Mach M (1997) The humoral immune response against human cytomegalovirus is characterized by a delayed synthesis of glycoprotein-specific antibodies. J Infect Dis 175:533–544
89. Schoppel K, Schmidt C, Einsele H, Hebart H, Mach M (1998) Kinetics of the antibody response against human cytomegalovirus-specific proteins in allogeneic bone marrow transplant recipients. J Infect Dis 178:1233–1243
90. Baccard-longere M, Freimuth F, Cointe D, Seigneurin JM, Grangeot-Keros L (2001) Multicenter evaluation of a rapid and convenient method for determination of cytomegalovirus immunoglobulin G avidity. Clin Diagn Lab Immunol 8:429–431
91. Lazzarotto T, Spezzacatena P, Pradelli P, Abate DA, Varani S, Landini MP (1997) Avidity of immunoglobulin G directed against human cystomegalovirus during primary and secondary infections in immunocompetent and immunocompromised subjects. Clin Diagn Lab Immunol 4:469–473
92. Lazzarotto T, Spezzacatena P, Varani S, Gabrielli L, Pradelli P, Guerra B, Landini MP (1999) Anticytomegalovirus (anti-CMV) immunoglobulin G avidity in identification of pregnant women at risk of transmitting congenital CMV infection. Clin Diagn Lab Immunol 6:127–129
93. van Zanten J, Harmsen MC, van der Giessen M, van der Bij W, Prop J, de Leij L, The TH (1995) Humoral immune response against human cytomegalovirus (HCMV)-specific proteins after HCMV infection in lung transplantation as detected with recombinant and naturally occurring proteins. Clin Diagn Lab Immunol 2:214–218
94. Shimamura M, Mach M, Britt WJ (2006) Human cytomegalovirus infection elicits a glycoprotein M (gM)/gN-specific virus-neutralizing antibody response. J Virol 80:4591–4600
95. Ohta A, Fujita A, Murayama T, Iba Y, Kurosawa Y, Yoshikawa T, Asano Y (2009) Recombinant human monoclonal antibodies to human cytomegalovirus glycoprotein B neutralize virus in a complement-dependent manner. Microbes Infect 11(13):1029–1036. https://doi.org/10.1016/j.micinf.2009.07.010
96. Britt WJ, Mach M (1996) Human cytomegalovirus glycoproteins. Intervirology 39:401–412
97. Schoppel K, Haßfurther E, Britt W, Ohlin M, Borrebaeck CAK, Mach M (1996) Antibodies specific for the antigenic domain 1 of glycoprotein B (gpUL55) of human cytomegalovirus bind to different substructures. Virology 216:133–145
98. Klein M, Schoppel K, Amvrossiadis N, Mach M (1999) Strain-specific neutralization of human cytomegalovirus isolates by human sera. J Virol 73:878–886
99. Cui X, Meza BP, Adler SP, McVoy MA (2008) Cytomegalovirus vaccines fail to induce epithelial entry neutralizing antibodies comparable to natural infection. Vaccine 26:5760–5766
100. Dörner T, Radbruch A (2007) Antibodies and B cell memora in viral immunity. Immunity 27:384–392
101. Wirtz N, Schader SI, Holtappels R, simon CO, Lemmermann NAW, Reddehase MJ, Podlech J (2008) Polyconal cytomegalovirus-specific antibodies not only prevent virus dissemination from the portal of entry but also inhibit focal virus spread within target tissues. Med Microbiol Immunol 197:151–158

102. Meyer H, Sundqvist VA, Pereira L, Mach M (1992) Glycoprotein gp116 of human cytomegalovirus contains epitopes for strain-common and strain-specific antibodies. J Gen Virol 73 (Pt 9):2375–2383
103. Spindler N, Rücker P, Pötzsch S et al (2013) Characterization of a discontinuous neutralizing epitope on glycoprotein B of human cytomegalovirus. J Virol 87(16):8927–8939
104. Urban M, Britt W, Mach M (1992) The dominant linear neutralizing antibody-binding site of glycoprotein gp86 of human cytomegalovirus is strain specific. J Virol 66(3):1301–1311
105. Burkhardt C, Himmelein S, Britt W, Winkler T, Mach M (2009) Glycoprotein n subtypes of human cytomegalovirus induce a strain-specific antibody response during natural infection. J Gen Virol 90(Pt 8):1951–1961
106. Cui X, Freed DC, Wang D et al (2017) Impact of antibodies and strain polymorphisms on cytomegalovirus entry and spread in fibroblasts and epithelial cells. J Virol 91(13):e01650–e01616
107. Maidji E, McDonagh S, Genbacev O, Tabata T, Pereira L (2006) Maternal antibodies enhance or prevent cytomegalovirus infection in the placenta by neonatal Fc receptor-mediated transcytosis. Am J Pathol 168(4):1210–1226
108. Ndjamen B, Devashish SJ, Fraser SE, Bjorkman PJ (2016) Charactrization of antibody bipolar bridging mediated by the human cytomegalovirus Fc reseptor gp68. J Virol 90(6):3262–3267
109. Kropff B, Burkhardt C, Schrott J et al (2012) Glycoprotein N of human cytomegalovirus protects the virus from neutralizing antibodies. PLoS Pathog 8(10):e1002999
110. Silva MC, Schröer J, Shenk T (2005) Human cytomegalvorius cell-to-cell spread in the absence of an essential assembly protein. Proc Natl Acad Sci U S A 102(6):2081–2086
111. Jacob CL, Lamorte L, Sepulveda E, Lorenz IC, Gauthier A, Franti M (2013) Neutralizing antibodies are unable to inhibit direct viral cell-to-cell spread of human cytomegalovirus. Virology 444:140–147
112. Digel M, Sampaio KL, Jahn G, Sinzger C (2006) Evidence for direct transfer of cytoplasmic material from infected to uninfected cells durin cell-associated spread of human cytomegalovirus. J Clin Virol 37:1): 10–1): 20
113. Longo LD, Reynolds LP (2009) Some historical scpects of understanding placental development, structure and function. Int J Dev Biol 54(2–3):237–255. https://doi.org/10.1387/ijdb.082774ll
114. Chavan AR, Griffith OW, Wagner GP (2017) The inflammation paradox in the evolution of mammalian pregnancy: turning a foe into a friend. Curr Opin Genet Dev 47:24–32
115. Gambel P, Hunziker RD, Wegmann TG (1984) Reproductive immunology and the placental barrier hypothesis. Asian Pac J Allergy Immunol 2(2):336–338
116. Beer AE, Sio JO (1982) Placenta as an immunological barrier. Biol Reprod 26:15–27
117. Benirschke K, Kaufmann P (1995) Pathology of the human placenta, 3rd edn. Springer, New York
118. Fisher S, Genbacev O, Maidji E, Pereira L (2000) Human cytomegalovirus infection of placental cytotrophoblasts in vitro and in utero: implications for transmission and pathogenesis. J Virol 74(15):6808–6820
119. Maidji E, Percivalle E, Gerna G, Fisher S, Pereira L (2002) Transmission of human cytomegalovirus from infected uterine microvascular endothelial cells to differentiating/invasive placental cytotrophoblasts. Virology 304:53–69
120. Saji F, Samejima Y, Kamiura S, Koyama M (1999) Dynamics of immunoglobulins at the feto-maternal interface. Rev Reprod 4:81–89
121. Radulescu L, Antohe F, Jinga V, Ghetie V, Simionescu M (2004) Neonatal Fc receptors discriminates and monitors the pathway of native and modified immunoglobulin G in placental endothelial cells. Hum Immunol 65:578–585
122. Simister NE (2003) Placental transport of immunoglobulin G. Vaccine 21:3365–3369
123. Kane SV, Acquah LA (2009) Placental transport of immunoglobulins: a clinical review for gastroenterologists who prescribe therapeutic monoclonal antibodies to women during conception and pregnancy. Am J Gastroenterol 104:228–233

124. Szlauer R, Ellinger I, Haider S, Saleh L, Busch BL, Knöfler M, Fuchs R (2009) Functional expression of the human neonatal Fc-receptor, hFcRn, in isolated cultured human syncytiotrophoblasts. Placenta 30:507–515
125. Leach JL, Sedmak DD, Osborne JM, Rahill B, Lairmore MD, Anderson CL (1996) Isolation from human placenta of the IgG transporter, FcRn, and localization to the syncytiotrophoblast. J Immunol 157:3317–3322
126. Ben-Hur H, Gurevich P, Elhayany A, Avinoach I, Schneider DF, Zusman I (2005) Transport of maternal immunoglobulins through the human placental barrier in normal pregnancy and during inflammation. Int J Mol Med 16:401–407
127. Englund JA (2007) The influence of maternal immunization on infant immune responses. J Comp Pathol 137:S16–S19
128. Malek A (2003) Ex vivo human placenta models: transport of immunoglobulin G and its subclasses. Vaccine 21:3362–3364
129. Simister NE (1998) Human placental Fc Receptors and the trapping of immune complexes. Vaccine 16(14/15):1451–1455
130. Moffett A, Loke YW (2004) The immunological paradox of pregnancy: a reappraisal. Placenta 25:1–8
131. Jabrane-Ferrat N, Siewiera J (2016) The up side of decidual natural killer cells: new developments in immunology of pregnancy. Immunology 141:490–497
132. Le Bouteiller P (2013) Human decidual NK cells: unique and tghtly regulated effector functions in healthy and pathogen-infected pregnancies. Front Immunol 4:404
133. Rosenstein DL, Navarette-Reyna A (1964) Cytomegalic inclusion disease. Am J Obstet Gynecol 15:220–224
134. Cochard AM, Tan-Vinh L, Lelong M (1963) Le placenta dans la cytomegalie congenitale. Arch Fr Pédiatr 20:35–46
135. Mostoufi-zadeh M, Driscoll SG, Biano SA, Kundsin RB (1984) Placental evidence of cytomegalovirus infection of the fetus and neonate. Arch Pathol Lab Med 108:403–406
136. Benirschke K, Mendoza GR, Bazeley PL (1974) Placental and fetal manifestations of cytomegalovirus infection. Virchows Arch B Cell Pathol 16:121–139
137. Monif GRG, Dische RM (1972) Viral placentitis in congenital cytomegalovirus infection. Am J Clin Pathol 58:445–449
138. Altshuler G, McAdams AJ (1971) Cytomegalic inclusion disease of a nineteen-week fetus. Am J Obstet Gynecol 15:295–298
139. Mühlemann K, Miller RK, Metlay L, Menegus MA (1992) Cytomegalovirus infection of the human placenta. Hum Pathol 23(11):1234–1237
140. Sinzger C, Müntefering H, Löning T, Stöss H, Plachter B, Jahn G (1993) Cell types infected in human cytomegalovirus placentitis identified by immunohistochemical double staining. Virchows Arch A Pathol Anat Histopathol 423:249–256
141. McDonagh S, Maidji E, Chang HT, Pereira L (2006) Patterns of human cytomegalovirus infection in term placentas: a preliminary analysis. J Clin Virol 35:210–215
142. Weisblum Y, Panet A, Zakay-Rones Z et al (2011) Modeling of human cytomegalovirus maternal-fetal transmission in a novel dicidual organ culture. J Virol 85:13204–13213
143. Tabata T, Petitt M, Fang-Hoover J, Zydek M, Pereira L (2016) Persistent cytomegalovirus infection in amniotic membranes of the human placenta. Am J Pathol 186(11):2970–2986
144. Hemmings DG, Kilani R, Nykiforuk C, Preiksaitis J, Guilbert LJ (1998) Permissive cytomegalovirus infection of primary villous term and first trimester trophoblasts. J Virol 72 (6):4970–4979
145. Hemmings DG, Guilbert LJ (2002) Polarized release of human cytomegalovirus from placental trophoblasts. J Virol 76(13):6710–6717
146. Gabrielli L, Losi L, Varani S, Lazzarotto T, Eusebi V, Landini MP (2001) Complete replication of human cytomegalovirus in explants of first trimester human placenta. J Med Virol 64:499–504

147. Liu T, Zheng X, Li Q, Chen J et al (2015) Role of human cytomegalovirus in the profileration and invasion of extravillous cytotrophoblasts isolated from early placentae. Int J Clin Exp Med 8(10):17248–17260
148. Hamilton ST, Scott G, Naing Z et al (2012) Human cytomegalovirus-induced cytokine changes in the placenta with implications for adverse pregnancy outcomes. PLoS One 7(12): e52899
149. Garcia AGP, Fonseca EF, De Souza Marques RL, Lobato YY (1989) Placental morpholoby in cytomegalovirus infection. Placenta 10:1–18
150. Parry S, Holder J, Strauss JF III (1997) Mechanisms of trophoblast-virus interaction. J Reprod Immunol 37:25–34
151. Rassa JC, Ross SR (2003) Viruses and toll-like receptors. Microbes Infect 5:961–968
152. Yagel S (2009) The developmental role of natural killer cells at the fetal-maternal interface. Am J Obstet Gynecol 201(4):344–350
153. Xiao J, Barcia-Lloret M, Winkler-Lowen B, Miller R, Simpson K, Guilbert LJ (1997) ICAM-1-mediated adhesion of peripheral blood monocytes to the maternal surface of placental syncytiotrophoblasts. Am J Pathol 150(5):1845–1860
154. Chan G, Stinski MF, Guilbert LJ (2004) Human cytomegalovirus-induced upregulation of intercellular cell adhesion molecule-1 on villous syncytiotrophoblasts. Biol Reprod 71:797–803
155. Compton T, Kurt-Jones EA, Boehme KW, Belko J, Latz E, Golenbock DT, Finberg RW (2003) Human cytomegalovirus activates inflammatory cytokine responses via CD14 and toll-like receptor 2. J Virol 77(8):4588–4596
156. Boehme KW, Guerrero M, Compton T (2006) Human cytomegalovirus envelope glycoprotein B and H are necessary for TLR2 activation in permissive cells. J Immunol 177:7094–7102
157. Chaudhuri S, Lowen B, Chan G, DAvey A, Riddell M, Guilbert LJ (2009) Human cytomegalovirus interacts with till-like receptor 2 and CD14 on syncytiotrophoblasts to stimulate expression of TNFα mRNA and apoptosis. Placenta 30:994–1001
158. Chan G, Hemmings DG, Yurochko AD, Guilbert LJ (2002) Human cytomegalovirus-caused damage to placental trophoblasts mediated by immediate-early-gene-induced tumor necrosis factor-α. Am J Pathol 161(4):1371–1381
159. Chan G, Guilbert LJ (2005) Enhanced monocyte binding to human cytomegalovirus-infected syncytiotrophoblast results in increased apoptosis via the release of tumour necrosis factor alpha. J Pathol 207:462–470
160. Chan G, Guilbert LJ (2006) Ultraviolet-inactivated human cytomegalovirus induces placental syncytiotrophoblast apoptosis in a toll-like receptor-2 and tumour necrosis factor-α dependet manner. J Pathol 210:111–120
161. Kovács IJ, Hegedüs K, Pál A, Pusztai R (2007) Production of proinflammatory cytokines by syncytiotrophoblasts infected with human cytomegalovirus isolates. Placenta 28:620–623
162. Chou D, Ma Y, Zhang J, McGrath C, Parry S (2006) Cytomegalovirus infecton of trophoblast cells elicits an inflammatory response: a possible mechanism of placental dysfunction. Am J Obstet Gynecol 194:535–541
163. Bácsi A, Aranyosi J, Beck Z, Ebbesen P, Andirkó I, Szabo J, Lampé L, Kiss J, Gergely L, Tóth F (1999) Placental macrophage contact potentiates the complete replicative cycle of human cytomegalovirus in syncytiotrophoblast cells: role of interleukin-8 and transforming growth factor-ß1. J Interf Cytokine Res 19:1153–1160
164. Tóth FD, Mosbor-Petersen P, Kiss J, Aboagye-Mathiesen G, Hager H, Juhl CB, Gergely L, Zdravkovic M, Aranyosi J, Lampe L, Ebbesen P (1995) Interaction between human immunodeficiency virus type 1 and human cytomegalovirus in human term syncytiotrophoblast cells coinfected with both viruses. J Virol 69(4):2223–2232
165. Pereira L, Maidji E, McDonagh S, Genbacev O, Fisher S (2003) Human cytomegalovirus transmission from the uterus to the placenta correlates with the presence of pathogenic bacteria and maternal immunity. J Virol 77(24):13301–13314

166. McDonagh S, Maidji E, Ma W, Chang HT, Fisher S, Pereira L (2004) Viral and bacterial pathogens at the maternal-fetal interface. J Infect Dis 190:826–834
167. Andrews JI, Griffith TS, Meier JL (2007) Cytomegalovirus and the role of interferon in the expression of tumor necrosis factor-related apoptosis-inducing ligand in the placenta. Am J Obstet Gynecol 197:608.e1–608.e6
168. Weisblum Y, Panet A, Zakay-Rones Z et al (2015) Human cytomegalovirus induces a distinct innate immune response in the maternal-fetal interface. Virology 485:289–296
169. Scott GM, Chow SS, Craig ME et al (2012) Cytomegalovirus infection during pregnancy with maternofetal transmission induces a proinflammatory cytokine bias in placenta and amniotic fluid. J Infect Dis 205(8):1305–1310
170. DeMeritt IB, Milford LE, Yurochko AD (2004) Anctivation of the NF-κB pathway in human cytomegalovirus-infected cells is necessary for efficient transactivation of the major immediate-early promoter. J Virol 78(9):4498–4507
171. Prösch S, Staak K, Stein J, Liebenthal C, Stamminger T, Volk HD, Krüger DH (1995) Stimulation of the human cytomegalovirus IE enhancer/promoter in HL-60 cells by TNFα is mediated via induction of NF-κB. Virology 208:197–206
172. DeMeritt IB, Podduturi JP, Tilley AM, Nogalski MT, Yurochko AD (2006) Prolonged activation of NF-κB by human cytomegalovirus promotes efficient viral replication and late gene expression. Virology 346:15–31
173. Boehme KW, Singh J, Perry ST, Compton T (2004) Human cytomegalovirus elicits a coordinated cellular antiviral response via envelope glycoprotein B. J Virol 78(3):1202–1211
174. Wang X, Huong SM, Chiu ML, Raab-Traub N, Huang ES (2003) Epidermal growth factor receptor is a cellular receptor for human cytomegalovirus. Nature 424:456–461
175. Isaacson MK, Feire AL, Compton T (2007) Epidermal growth factor receptor is not required for human cytomegalovirus entry or signalling. J Virol 81(12):6241–6247
176. Compton T (2004) Receptors and immune sensors: the complex entry pathof human cytomegalovirus. Trends Cell Biol 14(1):5–8
177. Maidji E, Genbacev O, Chang HT, Pereira L (2007) Developmental regulation of human cytomegalovirus receptors in cytotrophoblasts correlates with distinct replication sites in the placenta. J Virol 81(9):4701–4712
178. Tabata T, McDonagh S, Kawakatsu H, Pereira L (2007) Cytotroblasts infected with a pathogenic human cytomegalovirus strain dysregulate cell-matrix and cell-cell adhesion molecules: a quantitative analysis. Placenta 28:527–537
179. Schleiss MR, Aronow BJ, Handwerger S (2007) Cytomegalovirus infection of human syncytiotrophoblast cells strongly interferes with expression of genes involved in placental differentiation and tissue integrity. Pediatr Res 61(5):565–571
180. Rauwel B, Mariamé B, Martin H, Nielsen R, Allart S, Pipy B, Mandrup S, DEvignes MD, Evain-Brion D, Fournier T, Davrinche C (2010) Activation of PPARγ by human cytomegalovirus for de novo replication impairs migration and invasiveness of cytotrophoblast from early placenta. J Virol 84(6):2946–2954
181. Roth I, Fisher SJ (1999) IL-10 is an autocrine inhibitor of human placental cytotrophoblast MMP-9 production and invasion. Dev Biol 205:194–204
182. Yamamoto-Tabata T, McDonagh S, Chang HT, Fisher S, Pereira L (2004) Human cytomegalovirus interleukin-10 downregulates metalloproteinase activity and impairs endothelial cell migration and placental cytotrophoblast invasiveness in vitro. J Virol 78(6):2831–2840
183. LaMarca HL, Nelson AB, Scandurro AB, Whitley GSJ, Morris CA (2006) Human cytomegalovirus-induced inhibition of cytotrophoblast invasion in a first trimester extravillous cytotrophoblast cell line. Placenta 27:137–147
184. Pereira L, Maidji E (2008) Cytomegalovirus infection in the human placenta: maternal immunity and developmentally regulated receptors on trophoblast converge. Curr Top Microbiol Immunol 325:383–395

185. Schust DJ, Tortorella D, Seebach J, Phan C, Ploegh HL (1998) Trophoblast class I major histocompatibility complex (MHC) products are resistant to rapid degradation imposed by the human cytomegalovirus (HCMV) gene products US2 and US11. J Exp Med 188(3):497–503
186. Huddleston H, Schust DJ (2004) Immune interactions at the maternal-fetal interface: a focus on antigen presentation. Am J Reprod Immunol 51:283–289
187. Zhang Y, Zhao A, Wang X, Shi G, Jin H, Lin Q (2008) Expressions of natural cytotoxicity receptors and NKG2D on decidual natural killer cells in patients having spontaneous abortions. Fertil Steril 90(5):1931–1937
188. Tilburgs T, Evans JH, Crespo AC, Strominger JL (2015) The HLA-G cycle provides for both NK tolerance and immunity at the maternal-fetal interface. Proc Natl Acad Sci U S A 112 (43):13312–13317
189. Siewiera J, El Costa H, Tabiasco J et al (2013) Human cytomegalovirus infection elicits new decidual natural killer cell effector functions. PLoS Pathog 9(4):e1003257
190. Schust DJ, Tortorella D, Ploegh HL (1999) Viral immunoevasive strategies and trophoblst class I major histocompatibility complex antigens. J Reprod Immunol 43:243–251
191. Terauchi M, Koi H, Hayano C, Tayama-Sorimachi N, Karasuyama H, Yamanashi Y, Aso T, Shirakata M (2003) Placental extravillous cytotrophoblasts persistently express class I major histocompatibility complex molecules after human cytomegalovirus infection. J Virol 77 (15):8187–8195
192. Jun Y, Kim E, Jin M, Sung HC, Han H, Geraghty DE, Ahn K (2000) Human cytomegalovirus gene products US3 and US6 down-regulate trophoblast class I MHC molecules. J Immunol 164:805–811
193. Crespo A, Strominger JL, Tilburgs T (2016) Expression of KIR2DS1 by decidual natural killer cells increases their ability to control placental HCMV infection. Proc Natl Acad Sci U S A 113(52):15072–15077
194. Rovito R, Claas FHJ, Haasnoot GW et al (2018) Congenital cytomegalovirus infection: maternal-child HLA-C, HLA-E, and HLA-G affect clinical outcome. Front Immunol 8:1904
195. van Egmond A, van der Keur C, Swings GMJS, Scherjon SA, Claas FHJ (2016) The possible role of virus-specific CD8+ memory T cells in decidual tissue. J Reprod Immunol 113:1–8
196. Nigro G, Adler SP, LaTorre R, Best AM (2005) Passive immunization during pregnancy for congenital cytomegalovirus infection. N Engl J Med 353:1350–1362
197. Adler SP, Nigro G (2008) The importance of cytomegalovirus-specific antibodies for the prevention of fetal cytomegalovirus infection or disease. Herpes 15(2):24–27
198. Mussi-Pinhata MM, Pinto PCG, Yamamoto AY, BErencsi K, de Souza CBS, Andrea M, Duarte G, Jorge SM (2003) Placental transfer of naturally acquired, maternal cytomegalovirus antibodies in term and preterm neonates. J Med Virol 69:232–239
199. Nozawa N, Fan-Hoover J, Tabata T, Maidji E, Pereira L (2009) Cytomegalovirus-specific, high-avidity IgG with neutralizing activity in maternal circulation enriched in the fetal bloodstream. J Clin Virol 46(Suppl 4):S58–S63
200. La Torre R, Nigro G, Mazzoco M, Best Al M, Adler SP (2006) Placental enlargement in women with primary maternal cytomegalovirus infectio is associated with fetal and neonatal disease. Clin Infect Dis 43:994–1000
201. Schleiss MR (2006) The role of the placenta in the pathogenesis of congenital cytomegalovirus infection: is the benefit of cytomegalovirus immune globuline for the newborn mediated trough improved placental health and function? Clin Infect Dis 43:1001–1003
202. Pereira L, Maidji E, McDonagh S, Tabata T (2005) Insights into viral transmission at the unterine-placental interface. Trends Microbiol 13(4):164–174
203. Mandel B (1969) Neutralization of viral infectivity: characterization of the virus-antibody complex, including association, dissociation, and host-cell interaction. Ann N Y Acad Sci 13 (83):515–527
204. Liu X, Ye L, Bai Y, Mojidi H, Simister NE, Zhu X (2008) Activation of the JAK/STAT-1 signalling pathway by IFN-γ can down-regulate functional expression of the MHC Class I-related neonatal Fc Receptor for IgG. J Immunol 181:449–463

Epidemiology: The Influence of Socioeconomic Differences

3

Gabriele Halwachs-Baumann

The poor, we're told, will always be with us. If this is so, then infectious diseases will be, too—the plagues that the rich, in vain, attempt to keep at bay.
Paul Farmer 1999, *Infections and Inequalities: The Modern Plagues*

3.1 Infant Mortality as a Social Mirror

In the last 150 years, infant mortality decreased continuously. In the middle of the nineteenth century, infant mortality rate was about 160 per 1000 live births in England with remarkable differences between largely agricultural counties (rate 110) and largely industrial counties (rate 163). This rate declined until the middle of the twentieth century to a rate of about 20–30/1000 live births [1]. The same situation was shown for other European regions and the United States [2, 3]. Leading causes of death were atrophy, debility, and marasmus, followed by diarrhea and enteritis and, on the third place, bronchitis and pneumonia. The association of infant mortality with poverty and bad housing was evident [1, 3]. This situation has not changed, as shown in the World Health Statistics 2009. Globally, an estimated 37% of deaths among children under 5 occur in the first month of life, most in the first week. Countries making the least progress are generally those affected by high levels of HIV/AIDS, economic hardship, or conflict. The disease incidence could be reduced by improved water and sanitation supply. However, because the availability and use of proven interventions at community levels remain low, pneumonia and diarrhea still kill 3.8 million children under 5 each year [4]. Studies analyzing infant mortality in the Americas showed a continuous reduction of infant mortality from

G. Halwachs-Baumann (✉)
Department of Laboratory Medicine, Regional Hospital Steyr, Steyr, Austria
e-mail: gabriele.baumann@gespag.at

G. Halwachs-Baumann (ed.), *Congenital Cytomegalovirus Infection*,
https://doi.org/10.1007/978-3-319-98770-5_3

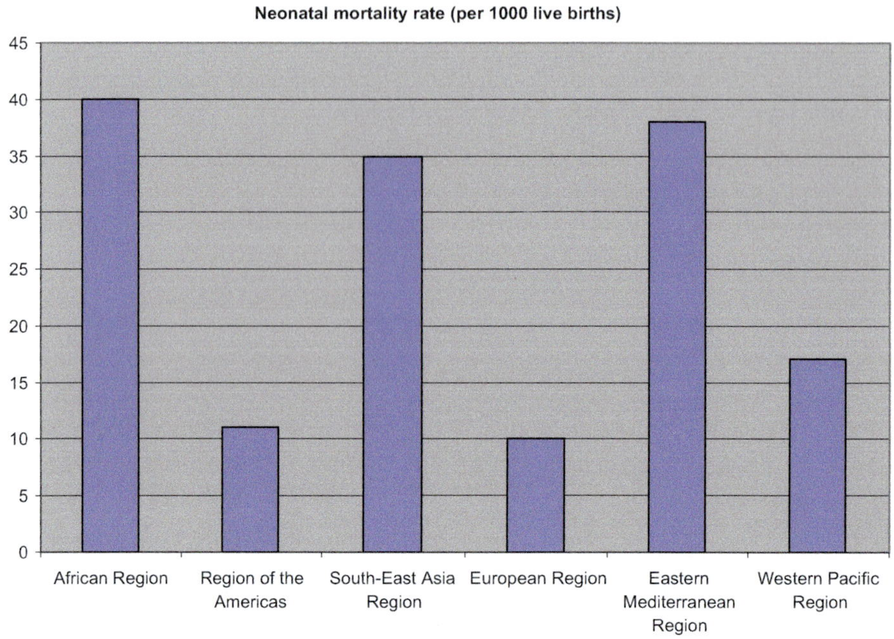

Fig. 3.1 Neonatal mortality rate

90.34 per 1000 live birth in 1955 to 31.31 in 1995, that is, a reduction of 65%. Not all of the countries of the region presented the same reduction. Paraguay, Guyana, Bolivia, and Haiti showed a decrease of 41–60%, while most of the countries (among others the United States) presented a reduction between 61–80%. A number of ten countries showed a decrease of more than 80%, with the highest percentage of reduction in Cuba (87.65%), Chile (88.33%), and Barbados (93.18%). One of the findings of this study is that social inequalities and inequality in health, two facts closely connected, persist in countries of the American Region. Government health expenditures in several countries are usually more beneficial for those better off than for the poor, although political will combined with effective public policies could move the focus of the expenditures of governments toward the poor (shown in Cuba, Chile, and Barbados), thus reducing infant mortality rate as indicator of the health conditions of the population [5].

Looking on the WHO data listed in the 2009 World Health Statistics, disparity between the WHO regions and income groups is remarkable (Figs. 3.1 and 3.2). Also the distribution of causes of death among children aged <5 years should be a matter of reflection. In the African Region, 61.2% of deaths among children aged <5 years are infectious diseases, compared to the regions of the Americas, Europe, and Western Pacific, where this percentage is < 30% (Table 3.1). The comparison of the income groups confirms the connection between poverty and infant mortality. In the lower-income group, infectious diseases as cause of death are six times higher than in the high-income group with a notable fissure between upper middle- and

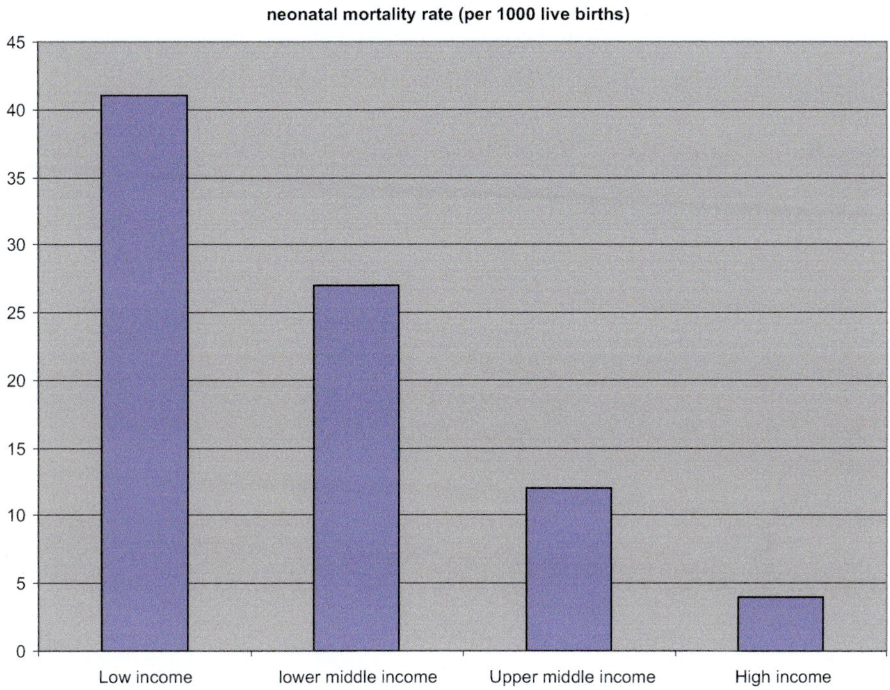

Fig. 3.2 Neonatal mortality rate

Table 3.1 Distribution of causes of death among children aged <5 years

WHO region	Infectious diseases (%)
African Region	61.2
Region of the Americas	26.3
Southeast Asia Region	39.5
European Region	29.7
Eastern Mediterranean Region	41.9
Western Pacific Region	23.2

Table 3.2 Distribution of causes of death among children aged <5 years

Income group	Infectious diseases (%)
Low income	56.3
Lower middle income	37.5
Upper middle income	32.9
High income	9.4

high-income groups (32.9% vs. 9.4%) (Table 3.2). Comparing only western industrialized nations, the United States show the highest rates in neonatal as well as in infant mortality rate, with slight differences depending on the source (Table 3.3). Looking closer to the situation in the United States, the highest infant mortality rate (8–8.99 and 9 or more) is seen in those states with the highest

Table 3.3 Infant mortality in western industrialized nations

	Source			
Nation	WHO (2004)	CIA (est. 2009)	UNECE (2006)	UNECE (2008)
Austria	3	4.42	3.6	3.7
Belgium	2	4.44	4	3.4
Cyprus	2	9.7	2.6[a]	
Czech Republic	2	3.79	3.3	2.8
Denmark	3	4.34	3.8	4
Finland	2	3.47	2.9	2.6
France	2	3.33	3.8	
Germany	3	3.99	3.8	3.5
Greece	3	5.16	3.7	3.5
Ireland	4	5.05	3.7	
Italy	3	5.51	4.2	3.7
Luxemburg	3	4.56	2.5	1.8
Netherlands	3	4.73	4.4	3.8
Norway	2	3.58	3.2	2.7
Portugal	3	4.78	3.3	
United Kingdom	3	4.85	5	
Switzerland	3	4.18	4.4	4
Sweden	2	2.72	2.8	2.5
Spain	2	4.21	3.8	3.5
Slovenia	2	4.25	3.4	2.1
Canada	3	5.04		
United States	4	6.22	6.7	
Australia	3	4.75		

WHO, neonatal mortality rate, deaths during the first 28 days of life per 1000 live births
CIA and UNECE, infant mortality rate, number of deaths of infants under 1 year old in a given year per 1000 live births in the same year
[a]Cyprus: Data cover only the area controlled by the Republic of Cyprus

percentage of Black or African American population and the highest percentage of poverty [6–8]. (Interestingly plotting these data in a map of the United States, the border between the Union and the Confederate States of America—the symbolic Mason-Dixon line—appears to resurface.)

There are a number of publications showing the significant race and ethnic difference in infant, neonatal, and postneonatal mortality. In African American infant, mortality rates are twice as high as for White infants, and the rates are rising. Maternal education and family income are inversely related to infant mortality rate; minority concentration and female divorce rates are positively associated with infant mortality [9–17]. The leading cause of death among Black infants was prematurity and low birth weight [7, 11, 14, 18]. Even children of Black college-educated parents have a higher mortality risk than similar White infants because of their higher rates of low birth weight. Black infants of this population are three times as likely as White infants to die of causes attributable to perinatal events, including prematurity.

Excluding low-birth-weight infants, the mortality rates of Black and White infants in this identical social class are equal [19, 20]. Interestingly, a study performed in New York City showed that Black very low-birth-weight (VLBW) neonates were more likely to be born at hospitals with higher neonatal mortality rates compared to White VLBW infants. This disparity in health-care providing is one explanation for the higher mortality rate in Black infants and explains one fourth of Black/White disparity. Another one is the higher percentage of Black VLBW infants compared to White VLBW infants (45.5% vs. 19.2% of all VLBW births) and that Black VLBW neonates are more likely to be born at lower birth weights within the VLBW category [21]. The association of deprivation with very preterm birth rate is not a sole phenomenon in the United States. Also in other industrialized countries, this connection is seen [22]. So in the United Kingdom, in deprived areas, the number of low gestational age, low birth weight, and low birth weight for gestational age is about twice as high compared to less deprived areas. Nevertheless, provision of care is equal between the various areas [23]. In the context of increasing preterm deliveries and low birth weight, the observations in Brazilian birth cohorts are of interest. As for industrialized countries in this middle-income country, the number of preterm infants and VLBW neonates increased, thus keeping the infant mortality rate constant from 1982 to 2004. Misuse of medicalization, epidemiological transition, and changing of risk factors do account for this trend [24, 25]. As a result of the changes in science and society, viral-host relationships will continue to change, and in so doing, they will produce a continuum of new problems [26].

3.2 One Effect: Many Causes

Overall the most common causes of infant mortality are infections. In contrast to this statistics including the whole world in western industrialized countries, congenital anomalies and disorders related to short gestation and unspecified low birth weight (Table 3.4) are the main cause for infant mortality. Nevertheless, fetal growth restriction can have many causes, etiologically associated with maternal, fetal, and placental factors.

3.2.1 Maternal Etiology

In about 20–40% of pregnancies complicated with fetal growth restriction, hypertensive disorders (gestational and non-gestational) of the mother are present [27, 28]. As a consequence of this, the uteroplacental blood flow is decreased. This is also the case in diabetes, chronic renal disease, and autoimmune disease. Besides these maternal diseases, environmental risk factors for fetal growth restriction exist. Maternal nutrition, smoking, alcohol and drug consumption, adolescent pregnancies, multiple births, and a shortened interval between pregnancies are known to be associated with adverse perinatal outcomes [29]. Preterm labor is one of the most common causes for low birth weight. Although preterm labor is a

Table 3.4 Anomalies and disorders related to short gestation and unspecified low birth weight

Causes of death	Singh 1995		National Vital Statistics Reports 2007		Statistics Austria 2008		German Federal Statistical Agency 2008	
	Absolute	%	Absolute	%	Absolute	%	Absolute	%
Congenital anomalies	7.388	30.15	5.636	36.95	83	28.92	603	24.98
Sudden infant death syndrome	5.161	21.06	2.247	14.73	22	7.67	215	8.91
Disorders related to short gestation and unspecified low birth weight	4.054	16.54	4.610	30.22	73	25.44	605	25.06
Respiratory distress syndrome	2.520	10.28			1	0.35	23	0.95
Newborn affected by maternal complications of pregnancy	1.507	6.15	1.706	11.18			53	2.20
Newborn affected by complications of placenta, cord, and membranes	933	3.81					94	3.89
Accidents and adverse effects	914	3.73	1.054	6.91	1	0.35	120	4.97
Infections specific to the perinatal period	860	3.51			7	2.44	56	2.32
Pneumonia and influenza	580	2.37					15	0.62
Intrauterine hypoxia and birth asphyxia	587	2.40					60	2.49
Others					100	34.84	570	23.61
Total	24.504		15.253		287		2.414	

syndrome with multifactorial etiology and incompletely elucidated pathophysiology, infections of the mother are discussed as one puzzle piece. Several randomized clinical trials have assessed the role of bacterial vaginosis treatment in prevention of preterm labor. The inconsistent results of these trials suggest that other processes, possibly immunomodulation, may be important [30]. Besides bacterial vaginosis, genital viral infections can occur. Mainly herpes virus infections are reported. Cervical shedding of CMV during reactivation is well documented [31]. In an Australian study, the presence of CMV was associated with preterm birth [32], whereas this observation was not made in an Italian report [33]. Since CMV infection of the pregnant women must not be associated with the infection of the newborn as exemplified in Chap. 2, CMV might play a role in pregnancy complications and complications of the newborn despite congenital CMV infection. To elucidate the connection of CMV infection (either systemic or local) with these complications, further investigations are necessary.

3.2.2 Fetal Etiology

Aneuploidy (7–30%) and fetal malformation (22%) are the most common causes for fetal growth restriction [27, 28]. The third place in that list is kept by perinatal infections (5–10%). Organisms known to cause congenital fetal infections are summarized by the acronym TORCH, first suggested by Nahmias et al. [34]. This group includes toxoplasma, rubella, cytomegalovirus, and herpes simplex virus. In the last years, the incidence of congenital syphilis is described to increase not only in developing countries, with a burden of mother-to-child transmission at least equal to HIV [35, 36]. In endemic countries malaria and hepatitis B have to be included in the list of congenital infections, but also parvovirus, enteroviruses, varicella-zoster virus, influenza virus, vaccinia, Epstein-Barr virus, and *Listeria* can affect the fetus [37–40]. In a study investigating the incidence of viral infections in intrauterine fetal death, CMV DNA was found in 16%, parvovirus B19 in 13%, and herpes simplex 1/2 in 5% of cases [41]. Estimated incidences of maternal and chronic intrauterine and perinatal infections for the United States were given by Alford [42]. Congenital CMV infection is listed first with an incidence of 0.5–2.2% of fetus and 8–13% of infants $\leq$6 months. Congenital CMV infection is also described in other publications as the most common found infectious disease in newborns [43, 44]. Incidence of congenital rubella varies considerably between epidemic and interepidemic periods (0.4–3% vs. 0.05%). In the last years, vaccination against rubella according to a survey of the member countries in the World Health Organization reduced congenital rubella syndrome substantially [45–48]. Some countries have met the target for reducing the incidence of congenital rubella syndrome to $<$1 case per 100,000 births, whereas others have not. Cultural and economic diversities of the regions, including social factors, political will, and economic costs, are reasons for this [45]. As for other infections, migration caused increases of incidences that are a challenge for health policy.

It has to be mentioned that congenital infectious disease not only are causative for infant mortality but also for infant morbidity not resulting in the death of the child, but in lifelong sequelae.

3.2.3 Placental Etiology

The placenta, as the vector for all maternal-fetal oxygen and nutrient exchange, is a principal influence on birth weight. Mainly uteroplacental blood flow affects birth weight [49]. This uteroplacental blood flow can be affected by defective placental development during implantation, as it occurs when endovascular erosion by trophoblasts is inadequate [50–52]. Furthermore gross lesions of infarct and abruption and chronic inflammation can lead to malnutrition of the fetus and thus intrauterine growth restriction [49]. Villitis can be found in 7–15% of placentas from infants small for date or with preterm birth [53, 54]. Acute and chronic inflammation can be seen. More than 50% hematogenous infections of the placenta can be demonstrated [54, 55]. The acute inflammatory response is overwhelmingly due to *Listeria* monocytogenes. Other rare causes of acute villitis/intervillositis are maternal exposure to *Chlamydia psittaci*, *Coccidioides immitis*, *Escherichia coli*, and group B and other streptococci. The later one can result in fetal sepsis [54]. TORCH infections cause chronic villitis [56]. The overwhelming majority of infectious chronic villitis in the United States is due to cytomegalovirus and *Treponema pallidum* [57]. However, herpes simplex virus, occasionally varicella zoster virus and poxviruses and rarely rubella virus in non-vaccinated populations may be responsible. Parasitic pathogens are uncommon in the United States [54]. Nevertheless the incidence of fetoplacental infection by *Toxoplasma gondii* was high in France [58] but could be reduced by the establishment of a screening and prevention program in 1978 [59, 60]. *Trypanosoma cruzi* (Chagas disease) as cause of chronic inflammatory placentitis is endemic in parts of South America [54]. Infection of the placenta must not implicate an infection of the fetus [61]. The isolated infection of the placenta as a result of maternal cytomegalovirus infection should be a matter of further investigations.

3.3 Epidemiology of Congenital CMV Infection

Cytomegalovirus infects people of all ages, races, and socioeconomic classes, throughout both the modernized and developing parts of the world. It is now well accepted that CMV is one of the most common viral causes of congenital infection. Nevertheless, the oft-cited 1% prevalence of congenital CMV infection has to be questioned. Meta-analysis considering diagnostic methods and the number of investigated cases gave more informative results. Overall, in the studies that assessed infection in all live-born infants, the combined birth prevalence of congenital CMV was 0.64% [62]. All studies showed a difference in the distribution of prevalence between Europe, North America, and other parts of the world (Table 3.5) [62–65]. Prevalence of congenital CMV is higher in a population with pre-existing positive CMV serostatus (0.81%) compared to women with negative pre-existing CMV serostatus (0.47%) (Tables 3.6 and 3.7). This increase of congenital CMV birth prevalence with maternal seroprevalence was observed, regardless of whether the study populations were ascertained at birth or during the prenatal period

Table 3.5 Distribution of the prevalence of congenital CMV infection

Authors	Region	Estimated prevalence	min–max
Halwachs-Baumann 2003 [63]	Europe	0.26%	0.04–0.49%
	North America	0.88%	0.22–2.20%
Kenneson 2007 [62]	North America		0.5–1.0%
Gaytant 2002 [64]	Europe		0.15–0.5%
	North America		0.42–1.4%

Table 3.6 Prevalence of congenitally CMV-infected children in preconceptionally seronegative pregnant women

Author	Year	Total number of seronegative pregnant women	Primary CMV infections in pregnant women	Congenitally CMV-infected children		
				Absolute (n)	Transmission rate (%)	Per cent of total number
Stagno et al [74]	1986	4692 (middle- or upper income group)	77	30	39	0.64
Ahlfors et al [66]	1982	1218	14	6	43	0.49
Nankervis et al [67]	1984	379	5	1	20	0.26
Kumar et al [68]	1984	1404	14	7	50	0.5
Stern and Tucker [69]	1973	270	11	5	45	1.85
Griffiths et al [70]	1980	1608	14	3	21	0.19
Grant et al [71]	1981	1841	13	5	38	0.27
Stagno et al. [72]	1982	1203	17	8	47	0.66
Stagno et al. [73]	1982	179	4	3	75	1.67
Gold and Nankervis*	1976	3000	8	4	50	0.13
Stagno et al [74]	1986	507 (low income group)	19	6	31.5	1.18
Yow et al [75]	1988	1940	21	7	33	0.36
Total		18,178	217	85		0.47

*Data from Ho M. Cytomegalovirus. Biology and infection. 2nd ed. Plenum Medical Book Company 1991

Table 3.7 Prevalence of congenitally CMV-infected children in preconceptionally seropositive pregnant women

Author	Year	Total number of seropositive pregnant women	Number of congenitally infected children	
			absolute	%
Stagno et al. [72]	1982	2330	20	0.86
Stagno et al. [76]	1977	208	7	3.37
Yow et al. [75]	1988	1959	7	0.36
Griffiths et al. [77]	1991	2000	5	0.25
Ahlfors et al. [66]	1982	3164	12	0.38
Nankervis et al. [67]	1984	710	15	2.11
Schopfer et al. [78]	1978	2032	28	1.38
Yamamoto et al. [79]	2001	452	9	1.99
Kamada et al. [80]	1983	1156	11	0.95
Total		14,011	114	0.81

[62, 64]. This observation may seem paradoxical, since one might expect that more seropositive women in a population would mean fewer pregnant women at risk for primary infection. Kenneson (2007) gives several explanations [62]:

A high-seroprevalence population means that there are more pregnant women at risk for reactivation. Even though reactivation is relatively infrequent for any given woman, on a population level, the number of affected women could be substantial. Cytomegalovirus seroprevalence depends on income and age, sociocultural factors, and sexual behavior [81, 82].

Seroprevalence may be high because there is a higher prevalence of risk behaviors in the population. So in a high-seroprevalence population, a pregnant woman has a higher likelihood of being exposed to someone who is CMV infected. Thus, seropositive pregnant women would have a higher risk of reinfection, and the relatively few seronegative pregnant women would have a higher risk of primary infection.

It was shown previously that reinfection with a different strain of CMV is an important cause of congenital CMV infection. Women preconceptionally seropositive for CMV who gave birth to congenitally CMV-infected infants showed in 62% acquired antibodies with new specificities [64]. So reinfection with another CMV strain is common [83]. These findings are in contrast to previous reports [84, 85] and might be due to improved diagnostic methods. In 1995 the report from the National Congenital Cytomegalovirus Disease Registry identified on the basis of mothers' characteristics two separate subpopulations of infants who had acquired congenital CMV infection: One group of infants was born to mothers 25 years of age or younger who were primarily primiparous, received Medicaid, and had an equal racial mix. The other group consisted of infants born to mothers older than 25 years of age who were mostly multiparous, were not recipients of Medicaid, and most often were White. They concluded that there may be two different sources of infection. The older multiparous mothers may acquire CMV from their preschool-aged children who attend group day-care centers, and the low-income, primiparous mothers may acquire CMV sexually [86]. This hypothesis is supported by the findings of Fowler et al. (1993) [87]: the screening of two diverse newborn populations showed a significant increase of congenital CMV infection with younger maternal age at delivery at the public hospital, whereas this association was not observed at the private hospital [87]. Age, race, marital status, social class, and parity of the mothers are individually strongly associated with the prevalence of congenital CMV infection [87–92]. The profession of the mother is another risk factor for infection. Women delivering congenitally infected infants are more likely to be students, salespersons, childcare providers, or teachers, whereas women who worked in health-care professions collectively had a reduced risk [90]. This reduced risk among offspring of women working in health-care occupations could reflect enhanced recognition of hygiene, training in standard precautions, or another behavior that reduces infection risk [90]. The high risk of teachers and day-care providers might be due to the high prevalence of CMV shedding among normal children. Once again the prevalence of infection and viral excretion depends on age (the highest rate is among toddlers 12–24 months of age), race, socioeconomic status, place of residence, and hygienic practices of the group [93]. Concerning the transmission from an infected toddler to a pregnant woman as risk for the unborn child to be infected with CMV, the Centers for Disease Control and Prevention (CDC) Workgroup on Congenital CMV recommends informing on congenital CMV and instructing pregnant women in hygienic practices [94].

As for other infectious diseases, the risk for transmitting the infectious agent to the unborn depends on the pre-existing serostatus of the mother. A meta-analysis described the risk of transmission during primary infections of the mother with 32.3% [62] and 44.9% [63], respectively. Data concerning the risk of transmission during secondary infections of the mother are more discrepant. Pooled estimations are between 1.4% [62] and 19.9% [63]. Looking on the details, the risk of transmission in the context of secondary CMV infections of the mother is given by the included studies between 0% and 33.3%. These differences are presumably due to the differences in definition and diagnosis of secondary CMV infections. Since most of the pregnant women have no symptoms and virus shedding in pregnant women is common [73, 95, 96], the estimation of the correct incidence of secondary infections is difficult. In a large cohort study, it was shown that naturally acquired immunity results in a 69% reduction in the risk of congenital CMV infection in future pregnancies [97]. So the remaining risk of transmission can be supposed to be about 10–14%.

The importance of pre-existing humoral immune response to CMV is demonstrated by the reduced occurrence of symptoms in congenitally infected newborns born to seropositive mothers [73, 98]. However, severe symptoms due to congenital CMV infection after recurrent maternal infection have been described and seem to be more common than supposed previously [99–102]. One aspect of CMV infection of the mother not very well investigated is the association with miscarriage or stillbirth. Besides case reports only few prospective studies exist

Table 3.8 Transmission rate and pregnancy trimester (number of infected mothers/number of infected newborns)

Author	Year	First trimester	Second trimester	Third trimester
Monif et al. [104]	1972	0/0	2/2	2/2
Stern and Tucker [69]	1973	2/2	4/2	5/1
Stagno et al. [105]	1986	33/17	10/6	26/14
Bodéus et al. [106]	1999	25/9	49/22	49/38
Preece et al. [107]	1983	10/2	20/0	15/6

[99, 101, 103]. Whether the virus must be already transmitted to the fetus or infection of the placenta is effectual cannot be said yet.

In contrast to other intrauterine infections in the case of CMV, the transmission rate seems not to depend on gestational age (Table 3.8), although the literature is not consistent [105]. As mentioned before primary infection poses a 30%–45% risk of intrauterine transmission, and adverse outcome is more likely when infection occurs within the first half of gestation [108, 109].

3.3.1 Congenital CMV and Virus Strains

Strain analysis in the context of congenital CMV infection is of interest concerning different questions. First of all sources of infection were identified by comparing CMV strains using polymerase chain reaction. So Murph et al. found in 1998 that mothers acquired CMV from community sources as childcare centers [110]. These findings confirmed prior observations of cytomegalovirus infection in newborns, showing that strains are related epidemiologically by point-source acquisition or transmission between individuals [111]. Second, investigations were performed to identify CMV strains predominantly vertically transmitted from mother to fetus. The most interesting polymorphic genes discovered to date are those encoding for viral envelope glycoproteins, mainly because their products are targets for neutralizing antibodies, often produced with a strain-specific pattern and involved in virus entry and cell-to-cell virus spread [112]. Glycoprotein B is an abundant envelope component. It is the major target for neutralizing antibodies and important for the entry of virions into cells and thus of major interest. Clustering the CMV strains by differences in the gB gene according to Chou and Dennison [113], the following distribution was found: genotype 1, 49%; genotype 2, 11%; genotype 3, 34%; and genotype 4, none [110]. These data are in accordance with other publications investigating the distribution of gB types within congenitally infected children, describing the gB type 1 as the dominant genotype in congenital CMV infection, followed by gB3, gB2, and gB4 [114–117]. This distribution differs from that observed in HIV/AIDS patients, where gB2 was the dominant genotype [117]; organ transplant patients, where gB3 was the dominant genotype; and bone marrow transplant patients, where gB1 was the dominant genotype, followed by gB2 [118]. No association between clinical outcome and gB type was seen

[119]. Interestingly in transplant recipients, the distribution of gB types differed between primary infection and reactivation. In the case of primary infection, gB type 3 was the most common virus strain, whereas in reactivation of CMV infection, gB type 2 was the most common [118].

Besides gB polymorphisms, variants in the UL73 gen (gN) are of interest. Changes within this gene were evident both at nucleotide and at amino acid levels [112]. There exist four gN types. All of them can cause congenital infection, with the following distribution: gN 1, 23%; gN 2, 1.1%; gN 3, 12.9%; and gN4, 62.4% [120]. As it was observed for the gB types, the distribution of the gN types differed between congenitally CMV-infected infants and other populations [112]. Considering the chronic outcome of congenital CMV infection, the gN1 variant is statistically significant more often associated with favorable chronic outcome [112, 120]. Recent data suggest that the CMV gN genotypes might be markers for virulence of CMV wild-type strains and a discriminating factor for selection of CMV-infected newborns who are at risk of developing sequelae. This hypothesis is based on the notice that newborns congenitally infected with CMV fall into two subpopulations: The first with no symptoms at birth, negative instrumental findings, and a favorable long-term outcome is significantly associated with gN-1 and gN-3a genotypes. The second group with symptoms at birth, abnormal imaging results, and sequelae was associated with gN-4 genotypes [121].

Last but not least, the polymorphism of virus strains is of interest in the context of secondary infections. Since transmission of the virus as a result of a secondary infection of the mother occurs not uncommonly, the question whether it is an endogenous or an exogenous reinfection is essential for the development of preventive strategies. In most of the cases of intrauterine transmission despite preconceptional existing immunity, the women acquired new antibody specificities. Although naturally acquired immunity results in a 69% reduction in the risk of congenital CMV infection in future pregnancies [122], reinfection with a different strain of CMV seems to be the major cause for secondary CMV infection [123]. In highly immune populations, 70%–80% of all infants with congenital HCMV infections are born to women undergoing nonprimary infection during pregnancy. This is even more striking in Africa, Asia, and South America, where maternal immunity to HCMV is often more than 95% in women of childbearing age and rates of congenital HCMV infections are often higher than in most other regions of the world [124]. Nevertheless, interpreting these results, comorbidities like HIV or malaria, socioeconomic status, and hygiene standard, factors known to support infections with CMV, have to be considered.

References

1. Aykroyd WR, Kevany JP (1973) Mortality in infancy and early childhood in Ireland, Scotland and England and Wales 1871–1970. Ecol Food Nutr 2:11–19
2. Moring B (1998) Motherhood, mild, and money. Infant mortality in pre-industrial finland. Soc Hist Med 11(2):177–196

3. Lee KS (2007) Infant mortality decline in the late 19th and early 20th centuries. Perspect Biol Med 50:585–602
4. World Health Statistics. 2009. www.who.int/whosis/whostat
5. Schneider MC, Castillo-Salgado C, Layola-Elizondo E et al (2002) Trends in infant mortality inequalities in the Americas: 1955–1995. J Epidemiol Community Health 56:538–541
6. McKinnon J. The black population: 2000. Census 2000 brief. 2001. http://ww.census.gov/population/www/cen2000/briefs.htlm
7. Mathews TJ, MacDorman MF (2007) Infant mortality statistics from the 2004 period linked birth/infant death data set. Natl Vital Stat Rep 55(14):1–31
8. http://www.census.gov/cgi-bin/saipe
9. Goldberg J., Hayes W., Huntley J. Understanding health disparities. The Health Policy Institute of Ohio. 2004
10. Singh GK, Yu SM (1996) US childhood mortality, 1950 through 1993: Trends and socioeconomic differentials. Am J Public Health 86:505–512
11. Singh GK, Yu SM (1995) Infant mortality in the United States: Trends, differentials, and projections, 1950 through 2010. Am J Public Health 85:957–964
12. Singh GK, Kogan MD (2007a) Widening socioeconomic disparities in US childhood mortality, 1969–2000. Am J Public Health 97:1658–1665
13. Singh GK, Kogan MD (2007b) Persistent socioeconomic disparities in infant, neonatal, and postneonatal mortality rates in the United States, 1969–2001. Pediatrics 119:e928–e939
14. Sims M, Sims TL, Bruce MA (2007) Urban poverty and infant mortality rate disparities. J Natl Med Assoc 99(4):349–356
15. Huynh M, Parker JD, Harper S, Pamuk E, Schoendorf KC (2005) Contextual effect of income inequality on birth outcomes. Int J Epidemiol 34:888–895
16. Bruckner TA, Saxton KB, Anderson E, Goldman S, Gould JB (2009) Prom paradox to disparity: Trends in neonatal death in very low birth weight non-hispanic black and white infants, 1989–2004. J Pediatr 155:482–487
17. Dominguez TP (2008) Race, racism, and racial disparities in adverse birth outcomes. Clin Obstetr Gynecol 51(2):360–370
18. Schrempf AH, Branum AM, Lukacs SL, Schoendorf KC (2007) The contribution of preterm birth to the black-white infant mortality gab, 1990 and 2000. Am J Public Health 97:1255–1260
19. Schoendorf KC, Hogue CJR, Kleinman JC, Rowley D (1992) Mortality among infants of black as compared with white college-educated parents. N Engl J Med 326:1522–1526
20. Wise PH, Pursley DM (1992) Infant mortality as a social mirror. N Engl J Med 326: 1558–1560
21. Howell EA, Hebert P, Chatterjee S, Kleinman LC, Chassin MR (2008) Black/white differences in very low birth weight neonatal mortality rates among New York City hospitals. Pediatrics 121:e407–e415
22. Craig ED, Thompson JMD, Mitchell EA (2002) socioeconomic status and preterm birth: New Zealand trends, 1980 to 1999. Arch Dis Child Fetal Neonatal Ed 86:F142–F146
23. Smith LK, Draper ES, Manktelow BN, Field DJ (2009) Socioeconomic inequalities in survival and provision of neonatal care: population based study of very preterm infants. BMJ 339: b4702
24. Barros FC, Victora CG, Barros AJD, Santos IS, Albernazu E, Matijasevich A, Domingues MR, Sclowith IK, Hallal PC, Silveira MF, Vaughan JP (2005) The challenge of reducing neonatal mortality in middle-income countries findings from three Brazilian birth cohorts in 1982, 1993, and 2004. Lancet 365:847–854
25. Costello A, Osrin D (2005) Epidemiological transition, medicalisation of childbirth, and neonatal mortality: three Brazilian birth-cohorts. Lancet 365:825–826
26. Weller TH (1998) Science, society, and changing viral-host relationships. Hosp Pract 30: 113–120
27. Maulik D (2006) Fetal growth restriction: the etiology. Clin Obstetr Gynecol 49(2):228–235

28. Hendrix N, Berghella V (2008) Non-placental causes of intrauterine growth restriction. Semin Perinatol 32:161–165
29. Ergaz Z, Avgil M, Ornoy A (2005) Intrauterine growth restriction – etiology and consequences: what do we know about the human situation and experimental animal models? Reprod Toxicol 20:301–322
30. Vidaeff AC, Ramin SM (2006) From concept to practice: the recent history of preterm delivery prevention. Part II: subclinical infection and hormonal effects. Am J Perinatol 23(2):75–84
31. Brabin BJ (1985) Epidemiology of infection in pregnancy. Rev Infect Dis 7(5):579–603
32. Gibson CS, Goldwater PN, MacLennan AH, Haan EA, Priest K, Dekker GA, for the South Australian Cerebral Palsy Research Group (2008) Fetal exposure to herpesviruses may be associated with pregnancy-induced hypertensive disorders and preterm birth in a Caucasian population. BJOG 115:492–500
33. Barbi M, Binda S, Caroppo S, Calvario A, Germinario C, Bozzi A, Tanzi ML, Veronesi L, Mura I, Piana A, Solinas G, Pugni L, Bevilaqua G, Mosca F (2006) Multicity Italian study of congenital cytomegalovirus infection. Pediatr Infect Dis J 25:156–159
34. Nahmias AJ, Josay WE, Naib ZM, Freeman MG, Fernandez RJ, Wheeler JH (1971) Perinatal risk associated with maternal genital herpes simplex virus infection. Am J Obstet Gynecol 110:825–837
35. Hawkes S (2009) Eliminating congenital syphilis – if not now then when? Sex Transm Dis 36(11):721–723
36. Woods CR (2009) Congenital syphilis – persisting pestilence. Pediatr Infect Dis J 28:536–537
37. Bale JF Jr (2002) Congenital infections. Neurol Clin N Am 20:1039–1060
38. Haun L, Kwan N, Hollier LM (2007) Viral infections in pregnancy. Minerva Ginecol 59: 159–174
39. Franca CM, Mugayar LRF (2004) Intrauterine infections: a literature review. Spec Care Dentist 24(5):250–253
40. Remington JS, Klein JO (1995) Infectious diseases of the fetus and newborn infant, 4th edn. W. B. Saunders Company, Philadelphia, PA
41. Syridou C, Spanakis N, Konstantinidou A, Piperaki ET, Kafetzis D, Patsouris E, Antsaklis A, Tsakris A (2008) Detection of cytomegalovirus, parvovirus B19 and herpes simplex viruses in cases of intrauterine fetal death: association with pathological findings. J Med Virol 80:1776–1782
42. Alford C (1982) An epidemiologic overview of intrauterine and perinatal infections of man. Mead Johnson Symp Perinat Dev Med 21:3–11
43. Abdel-Fattah SA, Bhat A, Ilanes S, Bartha JL, Carriongton D (2005) TORCH test for fetal medicine indications: only CMV is necessary in the United Kingdom. Prenat Diagn 25: 1028–1031
44. Deorari AK, Broor S, Maitreyi RS, Agarwal d, Kumar H, Paul VK, Singh M (2000) Incidence, clinical spectrum, and outcome of intrauterine infections in neonates. J Trop Pediatr 46:155–159
45. Spika JS, Wassilak S, Pebody R, Lipskaya G, Deshevoi S, Güris D, Emiroglu N (2003) Measles and rubella in the World Health Organization European region: diversity creates challenges. J Infect Dis 187(Suppl 1):S191–S125
46. Reef SE, Cochi SL (2006) The evidence for the elimination of rubella and congenital rubella syndrome in the United States: a public health achievement. Clin Infect Dis 43(Suppl 3): S123–S125
47. Centers for Disease Control and Prevention (CDC) (2005) Progress toward elimination of measles and prevention of congenital rubella infection – European region, 1990–2004. Morb Mortal Wkly Rep 54(7):175–178
48. Centers for Disease Control and Prevention (CDC) (2008) Progress toward elimination of rubella and congenital rubella syndrome – the Americas, 2003–2008. MMWR Morb Mortal Wkly Rep 57(43):1176–1179

49. Salafia CM, Charles AK, Maas EM (2006) Placenta and fetal growth restriction. Clin Obstet Gynecol 49(2):236–256
50. Ventolini G, Neiger R (2006) Placental dysfunction: Pathophysiology and clinical considerations. J Obstet Gynaecol 26(8):728–730
51. Salafia C (1997) Placental pathology of fetal growth restriction. Clin Obstet Gynecol 40(4): 740–749
52. Scifres CM, Nelson DM (2009) Intrauterine growth restriction, human placental development and trophoblast cell death. J Physiol 587(14):3453–3458
53. Nordenvall M, Sandstedt B (1990) Placental villitis and intrauterine growth retardation in a Swedish population. APMIS 98:19–24
54. Faye-Petersen OM (2008) The placenta in preterm birth. J Clin Pathol 61:1261–1275
55. Garcia AGP (1982) Placental morphology of low-birth-weight infants born at term. Contrib Gynecol Obstet 9:100–112
56. Altshuler G, Russel P (1975) The human placental villitides: a review of chronic intrauterine infection. Curr Top Pathol 60:64–112
57. Redline RW (2007) Villitis of unknown etiology: non-infectious chronic villitis in the placenta. Hum Pathol 38:1439–1446
58. Altshuler G (1977) Placentitis, with a new light on an old ToRCH. Obstet Gynecol Annu 6: 197–221
59. Thulliez P (1992) Screening programme for congenital toxoplasmosis in France. Scand J Infect Dis 84:43–45
60. Berger F, Goulet V, Le STrat Y, Desenclos JC (2009) Toxoplasmosis among pregnant women in France: risk factors and change of prevalence between 1995 and 2003. Rev Epidemiol Sante Publique 57(4):241–248
61. Hayes K, Gibas H (1971) Placental cytomegalovirus infection without fetal involvement following primary infection in pregnancy. J Pediatr 79:401–405
62. Kenneson A, Cannon MJ (2007) Review and meta-analysis of the epidemiology of congenital cytomegalovirus (CMV) infection. Rev Med Virol 17:253–276
63. Halwachs-Baumann G, Genser B (2003) Die konnatale Zytomegalievirusinfektion. Epidemiologie – Diagnose – Therapie. Springer, New York
64. Gaytant MA, Steegers AP, Semmekrot BA, Merkus HMMW, Galama JMD (2002) Congenital Cytomegalovirus infection: Review of the epidemiology and outcome. Obstet Gynecol Surv 57(4):245–256
65. Halwachs-Baumann G (2006) The congenital cytomegalovirus infection: virus-host interaction for defense and transmission. Curr Pharm Biotechnol 7:303–312
66. Ahlfors K, Ivarsson SA, Johnsson T, Svanberg L (1982b) Primary and secondary maternal cytomegalovirus infection and their relation to congenital infection. Analysis of maternal sera. Acta Paediatr Scand 71(1):109–113
67. Nankervis GA, Kumar ML, Cox FE, Gold E (1984) A prospective study of maternal cytomegalovirus infection and its effect on the fetus. Am J Obstet Gynecol 149:435–440
68. Kumar ML, Gold E, Jacobs IB, Ernhart CB, Nankervis GA (1984) Primary cytomegalovirus infection in adolescent pregnancy. Pediatrics 74(4):493–500
69. Tucker SH, M S (1973) Prospective study of cytomegalovirus infection in pregnancy. Br Med J 5:268–270
70. Griffiths PD, Campbell-Benie A, Heath RB (1980) A prospective study of primary cytomegalovirus infection in pregnant women. Br J Obstet Gynaecol 87:308–314
71. Grant S, Edmond E, Syme J (1981) A prospective study of cytomegalovirus infection in pregnancy. J Infect 3:24–31
72. Stagno S, Pass RF, Dworsky ME, Alford CA (1982d) Maternal cytomegalovirus infection and perinatal transmission. Clin Pbstet Gynecol 25(3):563–576
73. Stagno S, Pass RF, Dworsky ME, Henderson RE, Moore EG, Walton PD, Alford CA (1982b) Congenital cytomegalovirus infection. The relative importance of primary and recurrent maternal infection. N Engl J Med 306:945–949

74. Stagno S, Pass RF, Cloud G, Britt WJ, Henderson RE, Walton P d, Veren DA, Page F, Alford CA (1986b) Primary cytomegalovirus infection in pregnancy. Incidence, transmission to the fetus, and clinical outcome. J Am Med Assoc 256(14):1904–1908
75. Yow MD, Williamson DW, Leeds LJ, Thompson P, Woodward RM, Walmus BF, Lester JW, Six HR, Griffiths PD (1988) Epidemiologic characteristics of cytomegalovirus infection in mothers and their infants. Am J Obstet Gynecol 158:1189–1195
76. Stagno S, Reynolds DW, Huang ES, Thames SD, Smith RJ, Alford CA (1977) Congenital cytomegalovirus infection: Occurrence in an immune population. N Engl J Med 296:1254–1258
77. Griffiths PD, Baboonian C, Rutter D, Peckham C (1991) Congenital and maternal cytomegalovirus infections in a London population. Br J Obstet Gynaecol 98:135–140
78. Schopfer K, Lauber E, Krech U (1978) Congenital cytomegalovirus infection in newborn infants of mothers infected before pregnancy. Arch Dis Child 53:536–539
79. Yamamoto AY, Mussi-Pinhata MM, Cristina P, Pinto G, Figueiredo LT, Jorge SM (2001) Congenital cytomegalovirus infection in preterm and full-term newborn infants from a population with a high seroprevalence rate. Pediatr Infect Dis J 20(2):188–192
80. Kamada M, Komori A, Chiba S, Nakao T (1983) A prospective study of congenital cytomegalovirus infection in Japan. Scand J Infect Dis 15(3):227–232
81. Staras SAS, Dollard SC, Radford KW, Flanders WD, Fass RF, Cannon MJ (2006) Seroprevalence of cytomegalovirus infection in the United States, 1988–1994. Clin Infect Dis 43: 1143–1151
82. Chandler SH, Alexander ER, Holmes KK (1985) Epidemiology of cytomegaloviral infection in a heterogeneous population of pregnant women. J Infect Dis 152(2):249–256
83. Novak Z, Ross SA, Patro RK, Pati SK, Kumbla RA, Brice S, Boppana SB (2008) Cytomegalovirus strain diversity in seropositive women. J Clin Microbiol 46(3):882–886
84. Stagno S, Reynolds DW, Lakeman A, Charamella LJ, Alford CA (1973) Congenital cytomegalovirus infection: consecutive occurrence due to viruses with similar antigenic compositions. Pediatrics 52(6):788–794
85. Huang ES, Alford CA, Reynolds DW, Stagno S, Pass RF (1980) Molecular epidemiology of cytomegalovirus infections in women and their infants. N Engl J Med 303(17):958–962
86. Istas AS, Demmler GJ, Dobbins JG, Stewart JA (1995) Surveillance for congenital cytomegalovirus disease: a report from the National Congenital Cytomegalovirus Disease Registry. Clin Infect Dis 20(3):665–670
87. Fowler KB, Stagno S, Pass RF (1993) Maternal age and congenital cytomegalovirus infection: Screening of two diverse newborn populations, 1980–1990. J Infect Dis 168:552–556
88. Preece PM, Tookey P, Ades A, Peckham CS (1986) Congenital cytomegalovirus infection: predisposing maternal factors. J Epidemiol Community Health 40:205–209
89. Pannuti CS, Vilas-boas LS, Angelo MJO, Carvalho RPS, Segre CM (1985) Congenital cytomegalovirus infection. Occurrence in two socioeconomically distinct populations of a developing country. Rev Inst Med Trop Sao Paulo 27(2):105–107
90. Murph JR, Souza IE, Dawson JD, Benson P, Petheram SJ, Pfab D, Gregg A, O'Neill ME, Zimmerman B, Bale JF (1998a) Epidemiology of congenital cytomegalovirus infection: maternal risk factors and molecular analysis of cytomegalovirus strains. Am J Epidemiol 147:940–947
91. Stagno S, Dworsky ME, Torres J, Mesa T, Hirsh T (1982a) Prevalence and importance of congenital cytomegalovirus infection in three different populations. J Pediatr 101(6):897–900
92. Larke RPB, Wheatley W, Saigal S, Cheresky MA (1980) Congenital cytomegalovirus infection in an urban Canadian community. J Infect Dis 142(5):647–653
93. Onorato IM, Morens DM, Marone WJ, Stansfield SK (1985) Epidemiology of cytomegaloviral infections: Recommendations for prevention and control. Rev Infect Dis 7(4):479–497
94. Ross ES, Dollard SC, Victor M, Sumartojo E, Cannon MJ (2006) The epidemiology and prevention of congenital cytomegalovirus infection and disease: activities of the Centers For Disease Control and Prevention Workgroup. J Women's Health 15(3):224–229

95. Shen CY, Chang SF, Yen MS, Ng HT, Huang ES, Wu CW (1993a) Cytomegalovirus excretion in pregnant and nonpregnant women. J Clin Microbiol 31(6):1635–1636
96. Shen CY, Chang SF, Chao MF, Yang SL, Lin GM, Chang WW, Wu CW, Yen MS, Ng HT, Thomas JC, Huang ES (1993b) Cytomegalovirus recurrence in seropositive pregnant women attending obstetric clinics. J Med Virol 41:24–29
97. Fowler KB, Stagno S, Pass RF (2003a) Maternal immunity and prevention of congenital cytomegalovirus infection. J Am Med Assoc 289(8):1008–1011
98. Fowler KB, Stagno S, Pass RF, Britt WJ, Boll TJ, Alford CA (1992) The outcome of congenital cytomegalovirus infection in relation to maternal antibody status. N Engl J Med 326: 663–667
99. Gaytant MA, Rours IIJG, Steegers EAP, Galama JMD, Semmekrot BA (2003) Congenital cytomegalovirus infection after recurrent infection. case reports and reviews of the literature. Eur J Pediatr 162:248–253
100. Boppana SB, Fowler KB, Britt WJ, STagno S, Pass RF (1999) Symptomatic congenital cytomegalovirus infection in infants born to mothers with pre-existing immunity to cytomegalovirus. Pediatrics 104(1):55–60
101. Ahlfors K, Ivarsson SA, Harris S (1999) Report on a long-term study of maternal and congenital cytomegalovirus infection I Sweden. Review of prospective studies available in the literature. Scand J Infect Dis 31:443–457
102. Morris DJ, Sims D, Chiswick M, Das VK, Newton VE (1994) Symptomatic congenital cytomegalovirus infection after maternal recurrent infection. Pediatr Infect Dis J 13:61–64
103. Tanaka K, Yamada H, Minami M, Kataoka S, Numazaki K, Minakami H, Tsutusumi H (2006) Screening for vaginal shedding of cytomegalovirus in healthy pregnant women using real-time PCR: correlation of CMV in the vagina and adverse outcome of pregnancy. J Med Virol 78: 757–759
104. Monif GR, Egan EA, Held B, Eitzman DV (1972) The correlation of maternal cytomegalovirus infection during varying stages in gestation with neonatal involvement. J Pediatr 80(1): 17–20
105. Stagno S, Pass RF, Cloud G, Britt WJ, Henderson RE, Walton PD, VEren DA, Page F, Alford CA (1986a) Primary cytomegalovirus infection in pregnancy. Incidence, transmission to fetus, and clinical outcome. J Am Med Assoc 256(14):1904–1908
106. Bodéus M, Hubinont C, Bernard P, Bouckaert A, Thomas K, Goubau P (1999) Prenatal diagnosis of human cytomegalovirus by culture and polymerase chain reaction. 98 pregnancies leading to congenital infection. Prenat Diagn 19:314–317
107. Preece PM, Blount JM, Glover J, Fletcher GM, Peckham CS, Griffiths PD (1983) the consequences of primary cytomegalovirus infection in pregnancy. Arch Dis Child 58:970–975
108. Stagno S, Pass RF, Dworsky ME, Alford CA (1982c) Maternal cytomegalovirus infection and perinatal transmission. Clin Obstet Gynecol 25(3):563–576
109. Ahlfors K, Ivarsson SA, Johnsson T, Svanberg L (1982a) Primary and secondary maternal cytomegalovirus infection and their relation to congenital infection. Acta Paediatr Scand 71:109–113
110. Murph JR, Souza IE, Dawson JD, enson P, Petheram SJ, Pfab D, Gregg A, O'Neill ME, Zimmerman B, Bale JF (1998b) Epidemiology of congenital cytomegalovirus infection: maternal risk factors and molecular analysis of cytomegalovirus strains. Am J Epidemiol 147:940–947
111. Souza IE, Gregg A, Pfab D, Dawson JD, Benson P, O'Neill ME, Murph JR, Petheram SJ, Bale JF (1997) Cytomegalovirus infection in newborns and their family members: polymerase chain reaction analysis of isolates. Infection 25:144–149
112. Dal Monte P, Pignatelli S, Rossini G, Landini MP (2004) Genomic variants among human cytomegalovirus (HCMV) clinical isolates: the glycoprotein N (gN) paradigm. Hum Immunol 65:387–394
113. Chou SW, Dennison KM (1991) Analysis of interstrain variation in cytomegalovirus glycoprotein B sequences encoding neutralization-related epitopes. J Infect Dis 163(6):1229–1234

114. Bale JF, Murph JR, Demmler GJ, Dawson J, Miller JE, Petheram SJ (2000) Intrauterine cytomegalovirus infection and glycoprotein B genotypes. J Infect Dis 182:933–936
115. Lukácsi A, Taródi B, Endreffy E, Bábinszki A, Pál A, Pusztai R (2001) Human cytomegalovirus gB genotype 1 is dominant in congenital infections in South Hungary. J Med Virol 65:537–542
116. Barbi M, Binda S, Caroppo S, Primache V, Didò P, Guidotti P, corbetta C, Melotti D (2001) CMV gB genotypes and outcome of vertical transmission: study on dried blood spots of congenitally infected babies. J Clin Virol 21:75–79
117. Trincado DE, Scott GM, White PA, Hunt C, Rasmussen L, Rawlinson WD (2000) Human cytomegalovirus strains associated with congenital and perinatal infections. J Med Virol 61:481–487
118. Meyer-König U, Vogelberg C, Bongarts A, Kampa D, Delbrück R, Wolff-Vorbeck G, Kirste G, Haberland M, Hufert FT, von Laer D (1998) Glycoprotein B genotype correlates with cell tropism in vivo of human cytomegalovirus infection. J Med Virol 55:75–81
119. Pignatelli S, Dal Monte P, Rossini G, Landini MP (2004) Genetic polymorphisms among human cytomegalovirus (HCMV) wild-type strains. Rev Med Virol 14:383–410
120. Pignatelli S, Dal Monte P, Rossini G, Lazzarotto T, Gatto MR, Landini MP (2003) Intrauterine cytomegalovirus infection and glycoprotein N (gN) genotypes. J Clin Virol 28(1):38–43
121. Pignatelli S, Lazzarotto T, Gatto MR, Dal Monte P, Landini MP, Faldella G, Lanari M (2010) Cytomegalovirus gN genotypes distribution among congenitally infected newborns and their relationship with symptoms at birth and sequelae. J Infect Dis 51:33–41
122. Fowler KB, Stagno S, Pass RF (2003b) Maternal immunity and prevention of congenital cytomegalovirus infection. JAMA 289(8):1008–1011
123. Boppana SB, Rivera LB, Fowler KB, Mach M, Britt WJ (2001) Intrauterine transmission of cytomegalovirus to infants of women with preconceptional immunity. N Engl J Med 344(18): 1366–1371
124. Britt WJ (2017) Congenital human cytomegalovirus infection and the enigma of maternal immunity. J Virol 91(15):e02392-16

Prospects and Obstacles of Diagnosis

4

Gabriele Halwachs-Baumann

Diagnosis of CMV infection is characterized by a numerousness of laboratory methods reflecting the difficulties aligned with the clinic relevant diagnosis of this infection. Generally the used methods can be divided into those detecting the virus itself or parts of it (CMV DNA or RNA assays, electron microscopy, virus culture) and those detecting the immunological reaction of the host after having been confronted with the virus (serological assays, detection of CMV-specific cellular immunity). Another classification of CMV assays would be the division in screening assays and confirmatory assays. In the context of congenital CMV infection, serological assays play an important role for screening and risk stratification. Polymerase chain reaction for the detection and quantification of CMV DNA is used for the confirmation of a CMV infection and for risk stratification. Nevertheless, since molecular biology-based methods have got easier to handle and cheaper and thus are used more generally, these methods are more and more used for screening purpose.

4.1 Screening for Congenital CMV Infection

4.1.1 Screening of the Mother

Screening strategies can be done with the object to diagnose active infection during pregnancy or to diagnose CMV infection in the newborn. The chosen strategy is mostly dependent on the available therapeutic interventions and clinical reasonable suspicion, respectively. So, maternal CMV screening is frequently performed in conjunction with prenatal ultrasound findings [1–3], as it is the case in TORCH

G. Halwachs-Baumann (✉)
Department of Laboratory Medicine, Regional Hospital Steyr, Steyr, Austria
e-mail: gabriele.baumann@gespag.at

G. Halwachs-Baumann (ed.), *Congenital Cytomegalovirus Infection*,
https://doi.org/10.1007/978-3-319-98770-5_4

testing. TORCH is an acronym for organisms known to cause congenital fetal infections, namely, toxoplasma, rubella, cytomegalovirus, and herpes simplex virus. From these infectious diseases, only testing for CMV was published to be necessary, at least in the United Kingdom [4]. In countries, which have an obligatory program for medical investigations during pregnancy and childhood, as it is the medical record book for pregnancy and early childhood in Austria, TORCH tests like toxoplasmosis and rubella are performed despite prenatal suspicion of intrauterine infection. Screening for CMV infection is not performed yet. The ultimate cause for this might be the accounts of screening for disease, as it was framed by Wilson and Junger in 1968 [5]. Ten articles were formulated, among other requirements that there should be an accepted treatment for patients with recognized disease and there should be a suitable test or examination.

So management of pregnancy in a woman who is shown to have experienced a primary or near primary infection is a controversy still on debate [6]. Since the late 1960s of the last century, a lot of work has been done, and although there are still diagnostic problems linked to CMV in pregnancy, great progress was made in this area. From the late 1970s to early 1990s, non-specific markers like total serum IgM levels were discussed as screening parameters [7–9]. These unspecific tests are now generally assessed as obsolete. The common sense forces now CMV-specific tests as CMV-specific IgG, CMV-specific IgM, and CMV IgG avidity.

The first question that should be answered by diagnostic test is the risk of the pregnant women to acquire a primary CMV infection. This can be answered by the preconceptional serostatus of the women. Those who are CMV IgG positive before conception have a lower risk for active CMV infection during pregnancy. Women seronegative for CMV within the 6 months before conception are susceptible to primary CMV infection. These women should be tested for CMV-specific immunoglobulins at least twice, i.e., during months 2 and 4 of pregnancy [10]. The diagnosis of primary CMV infection is straightforward if seroconversion to CMV-specific antibodies is detected [11]. For women whose prepregnancy serological status is unknown, the diagnosis of CMV infection is complex. The first problem is that even primary infections are asymptomatic in most women. Approximately 90% of women will not develop symptoms [12]. So, clinical symptoms as evidence for an acute CMV infection lack enough sensitivity and specificity, respectively. Screening all women for CMV-specific IgM is the most appropriate procedure to detect active or recent CMV infection [10, 11, 13]. There is currently some concern over the fact that different commercially available kits frequently yield discordant results, limiting their diagnostic value. Agreement between kits varies from 56% to 76% with sensitivity between 30% and 88% [14, 15]. This is due to heterogeneity of the extracted antigen panel (natural source, recombinant antigens), cross-reactivity with other herpes virus (first of all Epstein-Barr virus), the influence of rheumatoid factors, etc. [15–18]. CMV IgM screening is recommended as a first step of a diagnostic algorithm in pregnancy, if no preconceptional serostatus is available. Thus, highly sensitive CMV-IgM test associated with further serological methods is the most targeting strategy [19]. Furthermore, once produced, CMV-IgM may persist for 6 to 9 months [11]. So, interpretation of results needs a good knowledge of these influencing and interfering factors. Recently, false-positive IgM for CMV in pregnant women with autoimmune disease were described. Interestingly the presence of these false-positive CMV IgM in these women was associated with a poor pregnancy outcome [20].

Besides the abovementioned problems of interpretation, CMV IgM positivity is not always a sign of primary infections. Primary infection and reactivation can be difficult to differentiate, to date especially for cases where no previous serology is available. Supplementary assays are therefore recommended to confirm positive IgM results. Immunoblotting and immunofluorescence were developed to distinguish between specific and non-specific reactions. However, these assays did not gain vast usage because of lowered sensitivity and lack of automation [13, 21]. To engineer diagnostic tool for the differentiation of primary and secondary CMV infection and to verify positive CMV IgM results, the knowledge about the special time line of the maturation and the composition of the humoral immune response against CMV was essential. A delay of 50–100 days in the appearance of glycoprotein-specific antibodies was observed, whereas immunoglobulins directed against other CMV-specific antigens were promptly synthesized [22]. This maturation is essential for sufficient defense capacities of the humoral immune system [23, 24] and can be therefore used as prognostic and discriminatory assays.

During the last years, CMV IgG avidity testing turned out to be the most promising test for practical purpose [21]. In the meantime commercially available and in-house methods were investigated for their validation in the context of CMV diagnosis [25–29]. The unanimous conclusion was the usefulness of CMV IgG avidity in the differentiation between primary and secondary infection. CMV-specific IgG avidity index can be used for pregnant women without a history of CMV seroconversion [12, 13] and for women with positive results for both tests, CMV IgG and CMV IgM. Low-avidity IgG in pregnant women persists for approximately 17 weeks, with full maturation of the antibody occurring approximately 25 weeks after onset of symptoms [30, 31]. Determination of anti-CMV avidity at 6–18 weeks' gestation can identify all women who would have an infected fetus/newborn (100% sensitivity), whereas at 20–23 week's gestation, the sensitivity of the test was lower (62.5%). A combination of CMV IgG avidity and CMV IgM yields the best results (81%) [11, 13]. So, a diagnostic algorithm for CMV serology in pregnant women is recommended as shown in Fig. 4.1 [10, 21, 30, 32].

Detection of low CMV IgG avidity in specimens from pregnant women indicates that primary CMV infection has occurred within the past 18–20 weeks [32], whereas medium to high avidity indicates a primary CMV infection $\geq$1.5 months before [21]. If primary infection is diagnosed, prenatal diagnosis is recommended. It can be discussed whether CMV IgM alone should be used as screening, CMV IgG testing should be done not till a positive CMV IgM result was obtained, or CMV IgM and CMV IgG testing is done in parallel. Both strategies would lead to the same results, and which one is chosen depends more on organizatory and monetary reasons.

Besides the question "how to screen pregnant women," there exists the discussion whether all pregnant women should be screened or just those at risk. Cahill et al. [33] published a decision analytic and cost-effectiveness model to compare three

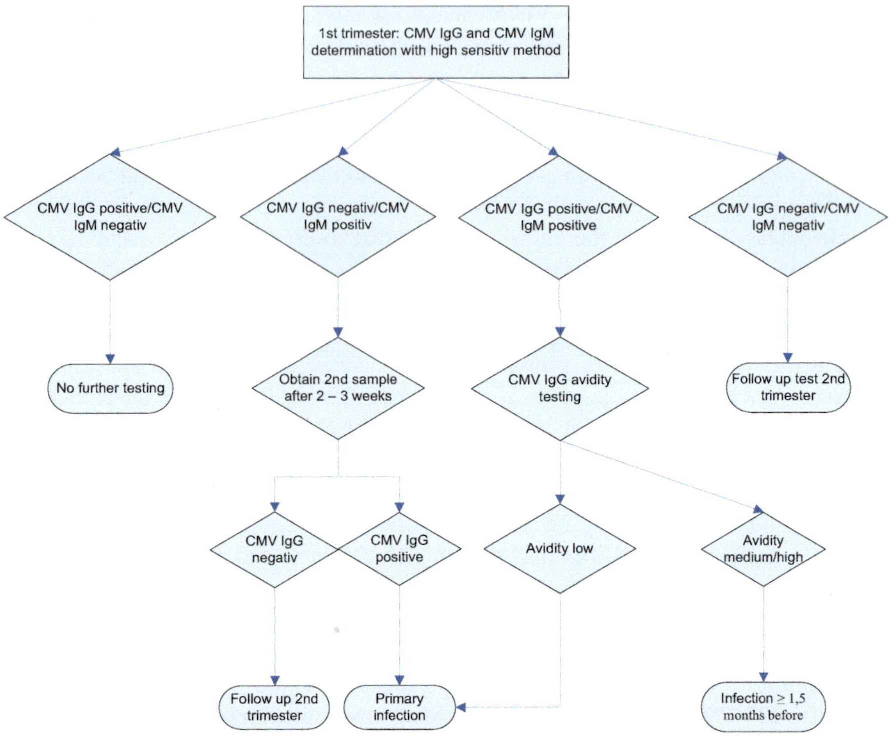

Fig. 4.1 Algorithm for the assessment of CMV infection in pregnancy

screening strategies for primary CMV infection with intention to treat. The three strategies were (1) screen all with intention to treat, (2) risk factor-based screening, (3) sonographic-based screening as a control group he used as (4) no screening or treating. They found out that universal screening is the most cost-effective strategy (cost and cost effectivity will be discussed in more detail in Chap. 7 of this book). A further aspect of prenatal screening is the increased awareness of this problem in the pregnant mother and thus benefit from preventive behavioral interventions. The statement of G. J. Demmler-Harrison in his keynote address at the Second International Congenital Cytomegalovirus Conference 2008 elucidates this topic [34] in an emotional and striking way, when he writes:

> Pregnant women welcome any knowledge that can help them have a healthy baby. Just ask them! They deserve to make an informed choice about their lifestyles and careers. But they feel betrayed, guilty, and angry, and some eve suffer paralyzing depression, when they give birth to a baby with congenital CMV disease, and later learn, from the internet or other sources besides their own trusted physicians and public health officers to whom they look for guidance, that their baby's congenitally acquired CMV disease potentially could have been prevented by an ounce of CMV awareness and three simple hygienic precautions: do not kiss toddlers on the mouth or face (give big hugs or kisses on top of the head instead), to not share

food, drink or utensils (refrain from "one for mommy and one for baby"), and wash hands carefully after changing diapers and wiping away saliva or nasal secretions.

There is no doubt in the scientific community that screening for primary CMV infections has more pros than cons. Nevertheless, I've got a notion that the problem of screening for secondary CMV infection during pregnancy is not even ignored. It is correct that the transmission rate to the unborn is lower in that situation, that the symptoms of the infected newborn if any are in most of the cases less serious, and that there exists no trusty screening (and therapeutic) strategy. The latter one seems to be the major reason why nobody touches on this problem. Only in Canadian guidelines, published 2010, diagnosis of secondary infection is mentioned. It is recommended that diagnosis of secondary infection should be based on a significant rise of IgG antibody titer with or without the presence of IgM and high IgG avidity. In cases of proven secondary infection, amniocentesis may be considered, but risk-benefit ratio is different because of the low transmission rate. The grading of this recommendation was III-C [35].

4.1.2 Screening of the Newborn

Screening the pregnant mother makes sense when therapeutic **and** preventive strategies are available. It has the disadvantage that congenital CMV infections in succession with secondary infections of the mother are not detected. Screening the newborns has the advantage that all congenitally infected newborns (those infected in the case of primary as well as in the case of secondary infections of the mother) are detected. This screening strategy has the disadvantage that the infection of the child still has progressed.

From a methodological point of view, screening of the newborn can be done by serological assays or by assays based on molecular biological techniques. Concerning testing for anti-CMV-IgM in the cord vein blood or serum of the child at the time of birth, the specificity is excellent. Nevertheless diagnostic sensitivity is between 22% and 69% (Table 4.1). Despite the differences due to methodological heterogeneity, the immaturity of the newborn's immune system is explanation of this lack of sensitivity. Even though serological tests are easy to perform and have a lot of

Table 4.1 Sensitivity and specificity of anti-CMV-IgM in the diagnosis of congenital CMV infection

Author	Year		Sensitivity	Specificity
Stagno et al. [36]	1985	Anti-CMV-IgM cord vein blood	69%	94.3%
Donner et al. [37]	1993	Anti-CMV-IgM serum newborn	69%	n.d.
Griffith et al. [38]	1982	Anti-CMV-IgM serum newborn	n.d.	100%
Nelson et al. [39]	1995	Anti-CMV-IgM serum newborn	22%	100%
Halwachs et al. [40]	2000	Anti-CMV-IgM cord vein blood	46%	100%
Naessens et al. [41]	2005	Anti-CMV-IgM cord vein blood	44%	n.d.

advantages for processing large numbers of samples, the low sensitivity makes them unusable as a screening method in the newborn [41].

More reliable than serological screening is the detection of the virus in neonatal specimen by virus culture or polymerase chain reaction (PCR). Traditional virus isolation from saliva or urine specimens in tissue culture is still considered the standard method for identification of infants with congenital CMV infection [42–44]. Since this method is time-consuming, alternatives were looked for. Real-time polymerase chain reaction technology does not require tissue culture facilities and is amenable to automation with the screening of large numbers of specimens at low cost [45]. Although both methods have a high sensitivity and specificity, in the last years, molecular-based methods have become more and more suitable for routine diagnosis and thus are now mainly replacing culture methods. Screening neonates for virus shedding has to mind two subjects. First, the tests must be done within the first 2–3 weeks after birth. Otherwise a discrimination between congenitally and peri- or postnatally acquired CMV infection cannot be done. That means that the detection of virus shedding within this time (far better to do the test at the time of birth or within the first postnatally week) is evidentiary for a congenitally acquired CMV infection. Second, cytomegalovirus load differs significantly in various body fluids of congenitally infected newborns. In urine the virus load can be 2–3 $\log_{10}$ higher than in cord vein blood [46]. So, urine is, despite problems with collecting procedures, the most reliable sample for the screening and diagnosis of congenital CMV infection. To reduce labor and consequently costs per test, screening urine pools for CMV DNA by nested PCR was evaluated. The authors concluded that urine pools (five samples each) and subsequent testing of the individual samples of a positive pool can be used to detect CMV-positive urines [47].

Two distinct newborn screening tests and programs exist in high-income countries. One system is the universal newborn hearing screening. This screening alone is insufficient to detect all CMV-infected infants because most infants with congenital CMV infection have normal hearing in the neonatal period [48]. The other system uses dried blood spot specimens collected on filter paper cards during the first week of life to conduct biochemical tests in centralized laboratories. The newborn blood spot screening (NBS) infrastructure was pioneered in the United States by Robert Guthrie in 1962 to screen for phenylketonuria. The filter cards for the sampling of the dried blood spots are still named after him—Guthrie card. Since 2000, the number of disorders included in NBS panels has expanded [49, 50]. Testing for CMV DNA in neonatal blood collected on filter paper has proved a valid means of diagnosis with both clinical and epidemiological relevance [51–54]. This screening approach is promising but still hampered by methodological incongruity [50, 55, 56] leading to different sensitivities (Table 4.2). External quality assessment of cytomegalovirus DNA detection on dried blood spots has shown discrepant results mainly in samples with low copies (10^2–10^3 copies/ml). Even in samples with a viral load of 8.8×10^4 copies/ml or higher, only 91% of participants gave correct positive results. Besides false-negative results, 9% of laboratories gave false-positive results [51]. These results show the great need of standardization of this method. Establishment of a universal standard would facilitate comparison of

Table 4.2 Sensitivity of CMV DNA PCR for the analysis of dried blood spots

Author	Year	Method	Sensitivity (%)
Soetens et al. [55]	2008	Manual extraction + conventional PCR	66
		EasyMAG extraction + real-time PCR	73
		Manual extraction + real-time PCR	82
		EasyMAG extraction + conventional PCR	45
Boppana et al. [45]	2010	Single-primer DBS PCR	28.3
		Two-primer DBS PCR	34.4
Barbi et al. [57]	2006	Not explained	99
Barbi et al. [58]	1996	Extraction with water/amplification of IE1	58
		Extraction with water/amplification of gp58	89
		Extraction with MEM/amplification of IE1	63
		Extraction with MEM/amplification of gp58	100
De Vries et al. [59]	2009	Method published by Barbi et al. 2000: Virus loads 5–4 $\log_{10}$ copies/ml	100
		Virus loads 4–3 $\log_{10}$ copies/ml	86
		Virus loads 3–2 $\log_{10}$ copies/ml	50

numerical results across various laboratories using different platforms or reagents [60].

The screening for congenital CMV infection in the newborn by PCR is not only impaired by the differences in detection limits of the various assays, leading to false-negative results. Sequence diversity in the glycoprotein B gene can complicate the detection of CMV too. False-negative results can be obtained by mutations within the probe hybridization sites [61]. These problems can also occur in CMV PCR targeting CMV polymerase and immediate-early genes [60] and are independent of the virus load in the sample. In addition to methodological problems, preanalytical interferences like delayed sample preparation can lead to false results [62]. So, interpretation of results presumes a good knowledge on the assets and drawbacks of the used method.

Nevertheless, there are so many pros to use Guthrie card for the screening of congenital CMV that great efforts should be made to standardize this method, above all increasing sensitivity and eliminating false-negative results.

4.2 Diagnosis of Congenital CMV Infection

4.2.1 Prenatal Diagnosis

After the suspicion of a primary infection in the pregnant women, two questions are to be considered with regard to the antenatal diagnosis of congenital CMV infection. The first question is whether the fetus is infected, and the second is whether the fetus is symptomatic and, if so, to what extent. The detection of CMV in amniotic fluid is said to be effective in differentiating uninfected from infected fetuses [63, 64]. In the guidelines on CMV congenital infection [44], amniocentesis is recommended concerning the following indications:

Pregnant women with clinical signs compatible with a primary CMV infection

Presence of ultrasound abnormalities compatible with a fetal CMV infection

Serologic suspicion of a recent infection after a CMV screening (despite the absence of an indication)

This amniocentesis should be performed in or after the 21st week of pregnancy and at least 6 weeks from the time of maternal infection. This is important to avoid false-negative results, since transplacental passage of the virus takes about 3 weeks, as shown by CMV infection of placenta explants [65], and due to renal immaturity of the fetus before 21 weeks of gestation, which prevents the elimination of the virus into the amniotic fluid [63, 66]. The presumption of the delay of virus transmission hampered by placental factors, as shown by in vitro experiments, is strengthened by in vivo observations. Sensitivity of prenatal diagnosis results increases from 50% to 76.2% and 91.3%, when <8, 9–12, and >13 weeks, respectively, elapse between the onset of maternal infection and the procedure [67]. Negative predictive values improve accordingly from 44.4% to 80% and 92.3% from the three time intervals, respectively. The presence of CMV should be determined by PCR. This method has a sensitivity and specificity of 90–98% and 92–98%, respectively, compared to virus isolation by cultivation on fibroblasts, which has only a sensitivity of 70–80% [44].

The possibility to achieve a sensitivity of 100% for the detection of CMV in the amniotic fluid is prevented by the fact that intrauterine transmission of CMV is characterized by an unpredictable delay [63, 68, 69]. This means that, while nearly all uninfected fetuses are identified, about 7–8% of infected fetuses were missed and thus scored as false negative. Apart from the most sensitive techniques used, the sensitivity of prenatal diagnosis may be increased by repeated sampling [70]. In the paper of Liesnard among 44 diagnosed infected pregnancies, 12 were diagnosed at the second sampling [71]. It must be mentioned, although rare, complications of amniocentesis may include fetal loss ($<1\%$), leakage of amniotic fluid, and vaginal bleeding [72].

Interpreting viral load in amniotic fluid is still discussed controversially. On the one hand, a correlation between CMV viral load in the amniotic fluid and outcome for the fetus is reported [32, 73–75]. In these papers the presence of $\geq 10^3$ genome equivalents predicts mother-child infection with 100% probability, and $\geq 10^5$ genome equivalents predict the development of a symptomatic infection. No conclusive explanation was given for positive PCR results of $<10^3$ genome equivalents, having an 81% probability of absence of infection in the fetus/newborn [73]. That means CMV was detected in the amniotic fluid but not in the fetus/newborn—findings leading to confusion, since no conclusive pathophysiological explanation can be given. In contrast to these reports, others find no association between viral load in the amniotic fluid and development of symptoms. Instead, the viral load in amniotic fluid seemed to be related to the time during the pregnancy when the amniocentesis was performed. This explanation is enhanced by the observation of an increase in the viral load between two consecutive amniocenteses [63]. To date it can be suggested that CMV load in amniotic fluid correlates with fetal clinical outcome but might also be dependent on other factors, such as the gestational age at the time of amniotic fluid sampling and the time elapsed since maternal infection [76].

Besides amniotic fluid, fetal blood drawn by cordocentesis can be used for prenatal diagnosis. These samples can be used for the determination of CMV-specific IgM and for quantification of viral load. Sensitivity and specificity of CMV IgM in the fetal blood is reported to be 55–57% and 100%, respectively [70], showing about the same results as in cord vein blood. About the same findings are reported for the determination of viral load in fetal blood. Sensitivity of antigenemia (i.e., detection of the virus-specific protein pp65 in leucocytes) is described to be 58%; of viremia, 55.5%; and of leukoDNAemia, 82.3% [67, 70]. As for amniocentesis, there are complications described following cordocentesis. The rate of fetal loss is 1.7–1.9%, thus about twice as high as described following amniocentesis. Although fetal loss often cannot be attributed solely to the procedure itself, the higher complication rate and the lower sensitivity and specificity of diagnosis CMV infection of the fetus make the investigation of fetal blood gained by choriocentesis less suitable, compared to the investigation of amnion fluid [72].

4.2.2 Neonatal Diagnosis

Diagnosis of congenital CMV infection is done by the detection of virus shedding in body fluids. This can either be urine, which shows the highest amount of virus load [46], saliva, or blood. If virus shedding is detected within 2–3 weeks postnatally, the diagnosis "congenital CMV infection" is assured. Besides the diagnostic approach, prognostic aspects are a matter of interest. Especially the risk assessment for the development of late-onset sequelae is an important feature. As for prenatal diagnosis, virus load was evaluated for its prognostic properties—with controverse results. No differences in median virus load (either urine or blood) between symptomatic and asymptomatic neonates and those developing sequelae and those developing no sequelae, respectively, were seen in one study [46], whereas others described significant differences in virus load between those children suffering from symptoms (at birth or later on) and those having an asymptomatic infection [77]. Since a wide range of CMV DNA load in symptomatic as well as in asymptomatic children is found, leading to overlapping results for virus burden in the groups, a more strict definition of symptoms and a higher number of included newborns lead to a more clear evidence. So, viral load as predictive marker for hearing loss development is described by some investigators [78–81]. This viral load correlates with other unspecific markers of active CMV infection, as elevated liver enzymes like ASAT and ALAT [80, 82]. CMV DNA detection in cerebrospinal fluid was positive only in those children with symptoms at birth or those children who developed sequelae [46, 83, 84]. Nevertheless, negative results cannot exclude the development of symptoms later on, but positive results seem to identify those newborns at risk for poor neurodevelopmental outcome [84]. Unspecific inflammatory markers like total protein and leukocytes in the cerebrospinal fluid seem to be as predictive for neurological damage in congenitally CMV infected children as CMV-specific parameters [46, 85].

Besides the initial diagnosis of congenital CMV within the neonatal period, it might be important to evaluate retrospectively whether or not a child with clinical problems as hearing deficits had an intrauterine infection with cytomegalovirus. Since 26–42% of children with sensorineural hearing loss (SNHL) diagnosed at the age of 4 had congenital CMV infection [86, 87] due to a retrospective dried blood spots analysis, this information about the etiology of SNHL might be important for therapeutic purpose. New insights in the pathophysiological principles of the slow progression of SNHL confirm the positive effect of ganciclovir therapy in congenitally CMV infected children [88–90]. Thus, an additional antiviral therapy in those children with (retrospective) diagnosed congenital CMV infection might have a beneficial effect on stopping progression.

References

1. Enders G, Bader U, Lindemann L, Schalasta G, Daiminger A (2001) Prenatal diagnosis of congenital cytomegalovirus infection in 189 pregnancies with known outcome. Prenat Diagn 21(5):362–377
2. Zafar U, Ong S, Gray J, Martin WM, Kilby MD (2006) The limitations of cytomegalovirus screening. Prenat Diagn 26:866–877
3. Gagnon A, Wilson RD, Allen VM, Audibert F, Blight C, Brock JA, Désilets VA, Johnson JA, Langlois S, Murphy-Kaulbeck L, Wyatt P (2009) Evaluation of prenatally diagnosed structural congenital anomalies. J Obstet Gynaecol Can 31(9):875–881
4. Abdel-Fattah SA, Bhat A, Illanes S, Bartha JL, Carrington D (2005) TORCH test for fetal medicine indications: only CMV is necessary in the United Kingdom. Prenat Diagn 25(11):1028–1031
5. Wilson JMG, Junger G (1968) Principles and practice of screening for disease. World Health Organization, Public Health Papers No. 34.
6. Demmler GJ (2005) Screening for congenital cytomegalovirus infection: a tapestry of controversies. J Pediatr 146:162–164
7. Mahon BE, Yamada EG, Newman TB (1994) Problems with serum IgM as a screening test for congenital infection. Clin Pediatr 33(3):142–146
8. El-Mekki A, Deverajan I V, Soufi S, Strannegard O, Al-Nakib W (1988) Specific and non-specific serological markers in the screening for congenital CMV infection. Epidem Inf 101:495–501
9. Alford CA, Schaefer J, Blankenship WJ, Straumfjord j V, Cassady G (1967) A correlative immunologic, microbiologic and clinical approach to the diagnosis of acute and chronic infections in newborn infants. N Engl J Med 277(9):437–449
10. Landini MP, Lazzarotto T (1999) Prenatal diagnosis of congenital cytomegalovirus infection: light and shade. Herpes 6:45–49
11. Lazzarotto T, Gabrielli L, Lanari M, Guerra B, Bellucci T, Sassi M, Landini MP (2004) Congenital cytomegalovirus infection: recent advances in the diagnosis of maternal infection. Hum Immunol 65:410–415
12. Collinet P, Subtil D, Houfflin-Debarge V, Kacet N, Dewilde A, Puech F (2004) Routine CMV screening during pregnancy. E J Obstet Gynecol 114:3–11
13. Lazzarotto T, Varani S, Spezzacatena P, Gabrielli L, Pradelli P, Guerra B, Landini MP (2000) Maternal IgG avidity and IgM detected by blot as diagnostic tools to identify pregnant women at risk of transmitting cytomegalovirus. Viral Immunol 13(1):137–141

14. Lazzarotto T, Guerra B, Lanari M, Gabrielli L, Landini MP (2008) New advances in the diagnosis of congenital cytomegalovirus infection. J Clin Virol 41:192–197
15. Genser B, Truschnig-Wilders M, Stünzner D, Landini MP, Halwachs-Baumann G (2001) Evaluation of five commercial enzyme immunoassays for the detection of human cytomegalovirus-specific IgM antibodies in the absence of a commercially available gold standard. Clin Chem Lab Med 39(1):62–70
16. Halwachs-Baumann G (2007) Recent developments in human cytomegalovirus diagnosis. Expert Rev Anti Infect Ther 5(3):427–439
17. Kraat YJ, Stals FS, Landini MP, Bruggeman CA (1993) Cytomegalovirus IgM antibody detection: comparison of five asays. New Microbiol 16(4):297–307
18. Daiminger A, Bäder U, Eggers M, Lazzarotto T, Enders G (1999) Evaluation of two novel enzyme immunoassays using recombinant antigens to detect cytomegalovirus-specific immunoglobulin M in sera from pregnant women. J Clin Virol 13:161 b–16171
19. Gentile M, Galli C, Pagnotti P, Di Marco P, Tzantzoglou S, Bellomi F, Ferreri ML, Selvaggi C, Antonelli G (2009) Measurement of the sensitivity of different commercial assays in the diagnosis of CMV infection in pregnancy. Eur J Clin Microbiol Infect Dis 28:977–981
20. De Carolis S, Santucci S, Botta A, Garofalo S, Martino C, Perrelli A, Salvi S, Degennaro VA, De Belvis AG, Ferrazzani S, Scambia G (2010) False-positive IgM for CMV in pregnant women with autoimmune disease: a novel prognostic factor for poor pregnancy outcome. Lupus 19:844–849
21. Mendelson E, Aboudy Y, Smetana Z, Tepperberg M, Grossman Z (2006) Laboratory assessment and diagnosis of congenital viral infections: Rubella, cytomegalovirus (CMV), varicella-zoster virus (VZV), herpes simplex virus (HSV), parvovirus B19 and human immunodeficiency virus (HIV). Reprod Toxicol 21:350–382
22. Schoppel K, Kropff B, Schmidt C, Vornhagen R, Mach M (1997) The humoral immune response against human cytomegalovirus is characterized by a delayed synthesis of glycoprotein-specific antibodies. J Infect Dis 175:533–544
23. Boppana SB, Britt WJ (1995) Antiviral antibody responses and intrauterine transmission after primary maternal cytomegalovirus infection. J Infect Dis 171:1115–1121
24. Boppana SB, Pass RF, Britt WJ (1993) Virus-specific antibody responses in mothers and their newborn infants with asymptomatic congenital cytomegalovirus infections. J Infect Dis 167:72–77
25. Prince HE, Leber AL (2002) Validation of an in-house assay for cytomegalovirus immunoglobulin G (CMV IgG) avidity and relationship of avidity to CMV IgM levels. Clin Diagn Lab Immunol 9(4):824–827
26. Curdt I, Praast G, Sickinger E, Schultess J, Herold I, Braun HB, Bernhardt S, Maine GT, Smith DD, Hsu S, Christ HM, Pucci D, Hausmann M, Herzogenrath J (2009) Development of fully automated determination of marker-specific immunoglobulin G (IgG) avidity based on the avidity competition assay format: application for Abbott Architect cytomegalovirus and toxo IgG avidity assays. J Clin Microbiol 47(3):603–613
27. Bodéus M, Goubau P (1999) Predictive value of maternal-IgG avidity for congenital human cytomegalovirus infection. J Clin Virol 12:3–8
28. Blackburn NK, Besselaar TG, Schoub BD, O'Connell KF (1991) Differentiation of primary cytomegalovirus infection from reactivation using the urea denaturation test for measuring antibody avidity. J Med Virol 33:6–9
29. Gutiérrez J, Piédrola G, del Carmen Maroto M (1998) Value of cytomegalovirus (CMV) IgG avidity index for the diagnosis of primary CMV infection. J Infect Dis 178:599–600
30. Munro SC, Hall B, Whybin LR, Leader L, Robertson P, Maine GT, Rawlinson WD (2005) Diagnosis of and screening for cytomegalovirus infection in pregnant women. J Clin Microbiol 43(9):4713–4718
31. Lazzarotto T, Spezzacatena P, Pradelli P, Abate DA, Varani S, Landini MP (1997) Avidity of immunoglobulin G directed against human cytomegalovirus during primary and secondary

infections in immunocompetent and immunocompromised subjects. Clin Diagn Lab Immunol 4(4):469–473
32. Maine GT, Lazzarotto T, Landini MP (2001) New developments in the diagnosis of maternal and congenital CMV infection. Expert Rev Mol Diagn 1(1):19–29
33. Cahill AG, Odibo AO, Stamilio DM, Macones GA (2009) Screening and treating for primary cytomegalovirus infection in pregnancy: where do we stand? A decision-analytic and economic analysis. Am J Obstet Gynecol 201:466.e1–466.e7
34. Demmler-Harrison GJ (2009) Congenital cytomegalovirus: public health action towards awareness, prevention, and treatment. J clin Virol 465:S1–S5
35. Yinon Y, Farine D, Yudin MH (2010) Cytomegalovirus infection in pregnancy. J Obstet Gynecol Can 32(4):348–354
36. Stagno S, Tinker MK, Elrod C, Fuccillo DA, Cloud G, O'Beirne AJ (1985) Immunoglobulin M antibodies detected by enzyme-linked immunosorbent assay and radioimmunoassay in the diagnosis of cytomegalovirus infections in pregnant women and newborn infants. J Clin Microbiol 21(6):930–935
37. Donner C, Liesnard C, Content J, Busine A, Aderca J, Rodesch F (1993) Prenatal diagnosis of 52 pregnancies at risk for congenital cytomegalovirus infection. Obstet Gynecol 82(4):481–486
38. Griffiths PD, Stagno S, Pass RF, Smith RJ, Alford CA (1982) Congenital cytomegalovirus infection: diagnostic and prognostic significance of the detection of specific immunoglobulin M antibodies in cord serum. Pediatrics 69(5):544–549
39. Nelson CT, Istas A, Wilkerson MK, Demmler GJ (1995) PCR detection of cytomegalovirus DNA in serum as a diagnostic test for congenital cytomegalovirus infection. J Clin Microbiol 33(12):3317–3318
40. Halwachs-Baumann G, Genser B, Danda M, Engele H, Rosegger H, Fölsch B, Maurer U, Lackner H, Truschnig-Wilders M (2000) Screening and diagnosis of congenital cytomegalovirus infection: a 5-y study. Scand J Infect Dis 32(2):137–142
41. Naessens A, Casteels A, Decatte L, Foulon W (2005) A serologic strategy for detecting neonates at risk for congenital cytomegalovirus infection. J Pediatr 146:194–197
42. Stagno S, Pass RF, Reynolds DW, Moore MA, Nahmias AJ, Alford CA (1980) Comparative study for diagnostic procedures for congenital cytomegalovirus infection. Pediatrics 65(2): 251–247
43. Stagno S, Reynolds DW, Tsiantos A, fuccillo DA, Long W, Alford CA (1975) Comparative serial virologic and serologic studies of symptomatic and subclinical congenitally and natally acquired cytomegalovirus infections. J Infect Dis 132(5):568–577
44. Coll O, BEnoist G, Ville Y, Weisman LE, Botet F (2009) Guidelines on CMV congenital infection. J Perinat Med 37:433–445
45. Boppana SB, Ross SA, Novak Z, Shimamura M, Tolan RW, Palmer AL, Ahmed A, Michaels MG, Sánches PJ, Bernstein DI, Britt WJ, Fowler KB (2010) Dried blood spot real-time polymerase chain reaction assays to screen newborns for congenital cytomegalovirus infection. J Am Med Assoc 303(14):1375–1381
46. Halwachs-Baumann G, Genser B, Pailer S, Engele H, Rosegger H, Schlak A, Kessler HH, Truschnig-Wilders M (2002) Human cytomegalovirus load in various body fluids of congenitally infected newborns. J Clin Virol 25:S81–S87
47. Paixao P, Almeida S, Gouveia P, Binda S, Caroppo S, Barbi M (2005) Diagnosis of congenital cytomegalovirus infection by detection of viral DNA in urine pools. J Virol Meth 128:1–5
48. Bale JF (2010) Screening newborns for congenital cytomegalovirus infection. J Am Med Assoc 303(14):1425–1426
49. Grosse SD, Dollard S, Ross DS, Cannon M (2009) Newborn screening for congenital cytomegalovirus: options for hospital-based and public health programs. J Clin Virol 465:S32–S36
50. Barbi M, Binda S, Caroppo S, Primache V (2006) Neonatal screening for congenital cytomegalovirus infection and hearing loss. J Clin Virol 35:206–209

51. Barbi M, MacKay WG, Binda S, van Loon AM (2008) External quality assessment of cytomegalovirus DNA detection on dried blood spots. BMS Microbiology 8:2. https://doi.org/10.1186/1471-2180-8-2
52. Kharrazi M, Hyde T, Young S, Amin MM, Cannon MJ, Dollard SC (2010) Use of screening dried blood spots for estimation of prevalence, risk factors, and birth outcome of congenital cytomegalovirus infection. J Pediatr 157(2):191–197
53. Neto EC, Rubin R, Schulte J, Giugliani R (2004) Newborn screening for congenital infectious diseases. Emerg Infect Dis 10(6):1069–1073
54. Yamagishi Y, Miyagawa H, Wada K, Matsumoto S, Arahori H, Tamura A, Taniguchi H, Kanekiyo T, Sashihara J, Yoda T, Kitagawa M, Ozono K (2006) CMV DNA detection in dried blood spots for diagnosing congenital CMV infection in Japan. J Med Virol 78:923–925
55. Soetens O, Vauloup-Fellous C, Foulon I, Dubreuil P, De Saeger B, Grangeot-Keros L, Naessens A (2008) Evaluation of different cytomegalovirus (CMV) DNA PCR protocols for analysis of dried blood spots from consecutive cases of neonates with congenital CMV infections. J Clin Microbiol 46(3):943–946
56. Binda S, Caroppo S, Didò P, Primache V, Veronesi L, Calvario A, Piana A, Barbi M (2004) Modification of CMV DNA detection from dried blood spots for diagnosing congenital CMV infection. J Clin Virol 30:276–279
57. Barbi M, Binda S, Caroppo S (2006) Diagnosis of congenital CMV infection via dried blood spots. Rev Med Virol 16:385–392
58. Barbi M, Binda S, Primache V, Luraschi C, Corbetta C (1996) Diagnosis of congenital cytomegalovirus infection by detection of viral DNA in dried blood spots. Clin Diagn Virol 6:27–32
59. de Vries JJC, Claas ECJ, Kroes ACM, Vossen ACTM (2009) Evaluation of DNA extraction methods for dried blood spots in the diagnosis of congenital cytomegalovirus infection. J Clin Virol 465:S37–S42
60. Thorne LB, Civalier C, Booker J, Fan H, Gulley ML (2007) Analytic validation of a quantitative real-time PCR assay to measure CMV viral load in whole blood. Diagn Mol Pathol 16(2):73–80
61. Nye MB, Leman AR, Meyer ME, Menegus MA, Rothberg PG (2005) Sequence diversity in the glycoprotein B gene complicates real-time PCR assays for detection and quantification of cytomegalovirus. J Clin Microbiol 43(10):4968–4971
62. Schäfer P, Tenschert W, Schröter M, Gutensohn K, Laufs R (2000) False-positive results of plasma PCR for cytomegalovirus DNA due to delayed sample preparation. J Clin Microbiol 38(9):3249–3253
63. Goegebuer T, Van Meensel B, Beuselinck K, Cossey V, Van Ranst M, Hanssens M, Lagrou K (2009) Clinical predictive value of real-time PCR quantification of human cytomegalovirus DNA in amniotic fluid samples. J Clin Microbiol 47(3):660–665
64. Grose C, Meehan T, Weiner C (1992) Prenatal diagnosis of congenital cytomegalovirus infection by virus isolation after amniocentesis. Pediatr Infect Dis J 11:605–607
65. Gabrielli L, Losi L, Varani S, Lazzarotto T, Eusebi V, Landini MP (2001) Complete replication of human cytomegalovirus in explants of first trimester human placenta. J Med Virol 64: 499–504
66. Gouarin S, Palmer P, Cointe D, Rogez S, Vabret A, Rozenberg F, Denis F, Freymuth F, Lebon P, Grangeot-Keros L (2001) Congenital HCMV infection: a collaborative and comparative study of virus detection in amniotic fluid by culture and by PCR. J Clin Virol 21:47–55
67. Revello MG, Gerna G (2004) Pathogenesis and prenatal diagnosis of human cytomegalovirus infection. J Clin Virol 29:71–83
68. Revello MG, Lilleri D, Zavattoni M, Furione M, Middeldorp J, Gerna G (2003) Prenatal diagnosis of congenital human cytomegalovirus infection in amniotic fluid by nucleic acid sequence-based amplification assay. J Clin Microbiol 41(4):1772–1774
69. Catanzarte V, Dankner WM (1993) Prenatal diagnosis of congenital cytomegalovirus infection: false-negative amniocentesis at 20 weeks' gestation. Prenat Diagn 13:1021–1025

70. Revello MG, Gerna G (2002) Diagnosis and management of human cytomegalovirus infection in the mother, fetus, and newborn infant. Clin Microbiol Rev 15(4):680–715
71. Liesnard C, Donner C, Brancart F, Gosselin F, Delforge ML, Rodesch F (2000) Prenatal diagnosis of congenital cytomegalovirus infection: prospective study of 237 pregnancies at risk. Obstet Gynecol 95(6):881–888
72. Grose C, Itani O, Weiner CP (1989) Prenatal diagnosis of fetal infection: advances from amniocentesis to cordocentesis – congenital toxoplasmosis, rubella, cytomegalovirus, varicella virus, parvovirus and human immunodeficiency virus. Pediatr Infect Dis J 8:459–468
73. Guerra B, Lazzarotto T, Quarta S, Lanari M, Bovicelli L, Nicolosi A, Landini MP (2000) Prenatal diagnosis of symptomatic congenital cytomegalovirus infection. Am J Obstet Gynecol 183:476–482
74. Lazzarotto T, Varani S, Guerra B, Nicolosi A, Lanari M, Landini MP (2000) Prenatal indicators of congenital cytomegalovirus infection. J Pediatr 137:90–95
75. Lazzarotto T, Gabrielli L, Foschini PM, Lanari M, Guerra B, Eusebi V, Landini MP (2003) Congenital cytomegalovirus infection in twin pregnancies: viral load in the amniotic fluid and pregnancy outcome. Pediatrics 12:e153–e157
76. Gouarin S, Gault E, Vabret A, Cointe D, Rozenberg F, Grangeot-Keros L, Barjot P, Garbarg-Chenon a, Lebon P, Freymuth F (2002) Real-time PCR quantification of human cytomegalovirus DNA in amniotic fluid samples from mothers with primary infection. J Clin Microbiol 40(5):1767–1772
77. Lanari M, Lazzarotto T, Venturi V, Papa I, Gabrielli L, Guerra B, Landini MP, Faldella G Neonatal cytomegalovirus blood load and risk of sequelae in symptomatic and asymptomatic congenitally infected newborns. Pediatrics 206, 117(1):e76–e83
78. Vauloup-Fellous C, Ducroux A, Couloigner V, Marlin S, Picone O, Galimand J, Loundon N, Denoyelle F, Grangeot-Keros L, Leruez-Ville M (2007) Evaluation of cytomegalovirus (CMV) DNA quantification in dried blood spots: retrospective study of CMV congenital infection. J Clin Microbiol 45(11):3804–3806
79. Boppana SB, Fowler KB, Pass RF, Rivera LB, Bradford RD, Lakeman FD, Britt WJ (2005) Congenital cytomegalovirus infection: association between virus burden in infancy and hearing loss. J Pediatr 146:817–823
80. Bradford RD, Cloud G, Lakeman AD, Boppana S, Kimberlin DW, Jacobs R, Demmler G, Sanchez P, Britt W, Soong SJ, Whitley RJ (2005) Detection of cytomegalovirus (CMV) DNA by polymerase chain reaction is associated with hearing loss in newborns with symptomatic congenital CMV infection involving the central nervous system. J Infect Dis 191:227–233
81. Walter S, Atkinson C, Sharland M, Rice P, Raglan E, Emery VC, Griffiths PD (2008) Congenital cytomegalovirus: association between dried blood spot viral load and hearing loss. Arch Dis Child Fetal Neonatal Ed 93:F280–F285
82. de Castro Romanelli RM, Magny JF, Jacquemard F (2008) Prognostic markers of symptomatic congenital cytomegalovirus infection. Braz J Infect Dis 12(1):38–43
83. Kapusta M, dzierzanowska D, Dunin-Wasowicz D, Milewska-Bobula B, Dobrzansky A, Wojda U, Swiatkowska E, Blaszczyk G (2001) Detection of cytomegalovirus in infant cerebrospinal fluid by conventional PCR, nested PCR and PCR-digene. Acta Microbiol Polonica 50(3):263–274
84. Troendle Atkins J, Demmler GJ, Williamson WD, McDonald JM, Istas AS, Buffone GJ (1994) Polymerase chain reaction to detect cytomegalovirus DNA in the cerebrospinal fluid of neonates with congenital infection. J Infect Dis 169(6):1334–1337
85. Jones CA, Isaacs D (1995) Predicting the outcome of symptomatic congenital cytomegalovirus infection. J Paediatr Child Health 31(2):70–71
86. Ross SA, Ahmed A, Palmer AL et al (2017) Newborn dried blood spot polymerase chain reaction to identify infants with congenital cytomegalovirus-associated sensorineural hearing loss. J Pediatr 184:57–61

87. Meyer L, Sharon B, Huang TC et al (2017) Analysis of archived newborn dried blood spots (DBS) identifies congenital cytomegalovirus as a major cause of unexplained pediatric sensorineural hearing loss. Am J Otolaryngol 38(5):565–570
88. Halwachs-Baumann G (2016) Congenital cytomegalovirus infection and hearing impairment. Clin Res Infect Dis 3(2):1029
89. Lackner A, Acham A, Alborno T et al (2009) Effect on hearing of ganciclovir therapy for asymptomatic congenital cytomegalovirus infection: four to 10 year follow up. J Lanryngol Otol 123(4):391–396
90. James SH, Kimberlin DW (2016) Advances in the prevention and treatment of congenital cytomegalovirus infection. Curr Opin Pediatr 28(1):81–85

Clinical Outcome: Acute Symptoms and Sleeping Hazards

5

Thorsten W. Orlikowsky

5.1 Relevance of Connatal CMV Infection for the Pediatrician and Neonatologist

Congenital cytomegalovirus (CMV) infection is the most common potentially disabling perinatal infectious disease and most common viral cause of congenital infections, present in high- as well as low-resource countries. If primary infection occurs in the developing fetus or neonate, consequences can be severe: As an important contributor to serious neurodevelopmental sequelae in children, CMV infection affects 1% of all life births [1].

Therefore, it is a major public health concern worldwide, since CMV infection causes mental delay, cerebral palsy, sensorineural hearing loss, and blindness. Even with antiviral therapy, the infectious sequelae often are irreversible. The magnitude of the problem seems to be underestimated, and little awareness exists in the medical field and in general public concerning disease burden and incidence. Congenital CMV infection has been the major cause of birth defects and childhood disorders in the United States: It is estimated that about 40,000 children (0.2–2% of all deliveries) are born with CMV, resulting in about 400 fatal cases each year [2]. In Europe, it is clearly shown as well that congenital CMV infection has a high epidemiological impact on diseases and cost [3].

T. W. Orlikowsky (✉)
Department of Neonatology, University Children's Hospital, Aachen, Germany
e-mail: torlikowsky@ukaachen.de

G. Halwachs-Baumann (ed.), *Congenital Cytomegalovirus Infection*,
https://doi.org/10.1007/978-3-319-98770-5_5

5.2 The Tip of the Iceberg

Across the globe, CMV seroprevalence varies both between and within countries. As a rule of thumb, lower socioeconomic groups have a higher incidence of CMV exposure, and resource-poor countries also have higher seroprevalence levels with infection (from 84 to 100% IgG-positive) frequently acquired early in life [4]. These epidemiological patterns have a direct impact on the incidence of congenital infection and disease: The classic high-risk setting for congenital CMV infection and particularly disease is where a seronegative mother becomes infected during pregnancy (in particular, during the first trimester) and transmits the virus to the fetus. In this situation, transmission to the fetus occurs in 30–35% of cases and congenital disease in around 10–15% of those born with congenital infection (reviewed in [5]). Large epidemiological studies from the United States have shown that only 10–15% of children with congenital CMV infection show clinical signs at birth, the rest are asymptomatic but at risk for neurodevelopmental sequelae later in life [6]. 60–90% with symptomatic infection, and 10–15% of those with asymptomatic infection, develop one or more long-term neurological sequelae and ophthalmologic abnormalities [1, 7, 8]. Current estimates indicate that approximately 8000 children are affected each year with some neurological sequelae related to in utero CMV infection, with an incidence far greater than that of Down syndrome (4000/year), fetal alcohol syndrome (5000/year), or spinal bifida (3500/year), making congenital CMV infection the most common cause of birth defects and childhood disabilities in the United States [6]. In populations from low-resource countries, most children will acquire a CMV infection during the first years of life, and the seroprevalence in children from high socioeconomic populations, breastfed for more than 6 months, is higher than in children breastfed for shorter periods. As a consequence of the variation in seroprevalence between countries, the prevalence of congenital CMV also varies [9].

5.3 Lucky Chance by Neonatal Immune Response

Since CMV, as member of the herpes virus family, has coevolved with its vertebrate hosts for more than 100 million years, and since it is a ubiquitous DNA virus with the capacity to establish lifelong latency in hosts, there is a complex balance, the usual outcome of which is a clinically inapparent, persisting infection. Viral shedding may persist for years after a primary infection and contribute to viral spread. CMV employs a multitude of strategies to modulate the host immune response, facilitating its persistence even in the face of a robust innate and adaptive immune response, which is not yet present prenatally and after birth. The level of cross talk between innate and adaptive immune cells that is required for the development of effective immunity is complex and pathogen-specific, involving host cellular (e.g., natural killer cells) and humoral (e.g., type 1 interferons) immune mechanisms. Both clinical and experimental evidence demonstrates that the immune system during pregnancy is skewed to elicit predominantly Th2 responses, thus altering host susceptibility to various pathogens. Cytokines, such as interleukin-10 (IL-10), IL-5, and IL-4, predominate at the materno-fetal interface of the placenta, which is essential for maintenance of pregnancy. It has been postulated that the microenvironment at the materno-fetal interface selectively downregulates Th1 responses in the fetus, resulting in decreased IFN-γ production. With respect to the neonatal immune system with its known deficiencies in innate (e.g., reduced natural killer cell functions and type 1 interferons) and adaptive immunity, this translates into a high susceptibility for viral replication, cellular alteration, and destruction.

5.4 Features of Symptomatic CMV Infection

The classic anamnestic history includes oligohydramnios, polyhydramnios, prematurity, intrauterine growth retardation, fetal ascites, hypotonia, or nonimmune hydrops [10]. Recent observations of the placenta show that CMV particularly infects amniotic membranes, impairs cytotrophoblast-induced lymphangiogenesis and vascular remodeling in the placenta, and arrests the correct development of human trophoblast progenitor cells, thus interfering with the earliest stages in the growth of new villi. This results in increased hypoxia, which ultimately contributes to restriction in fetal growth. Immunohistochemical and virological studies of placental tissues suggest that severe placental infection is associated with diffuse villitis and necrosis, consistent with functional impairment and possible consequent hypoxic cerebral damage. CMV infection also appears to persist in the amniotic epithelial cells and has been associated with increased expression of the anti-apoptotic proteins survivin and Bclx-l (reviewed in [5]).

Within the huge diversity of maternal reasons for intrauterine growth retardation (e.g., HELLP syndrome, maternal drug, or nicotine abusus), connatal CMV infection is rather uncommon. On the other side, severe growth retardation may be present in up to 50% of symptomatically infected neonates. In contrast, asymptomatic newborns very rarely are found either premature or growth retarded.

The classic clinical picture of cytomegalic disease is characterized by involvement of multiple organs, in particular the reticuloendothelial and central nervous system. Unspecific symptoms consist of poor feeding, lethargy, and thermal instability. Obvious clinical symptoms are jaundice, hepatosplenomegaly, and petechiae (Fig. 5.1). Neurological involvement includes microcephaly, hearing loss, blindness, seizures, hypotonia, and lethargy. The most severely affected infants have a mortality rate of about 30%. Deaths are usually due to hepatic dysfunction, bleeding with intracranial hemorrhage, disseminated intravascular coagulation, or secondary bacterial superinfections.

Infants with symptomatic CMV infection may be at increased risk for congenital malformations such as inguinal hernia in males, high-arched palate, defective enamelization of the deciduous teeth, hydrocephalus, clasp thumb deformity, and clubfoot (Leung). Whereas clinical signs due to abnormalities of the reticuloendothelial system are mostly transient, neurological deficits and damage either are evident at birth and typically persist for life or tend to become fully apparent in

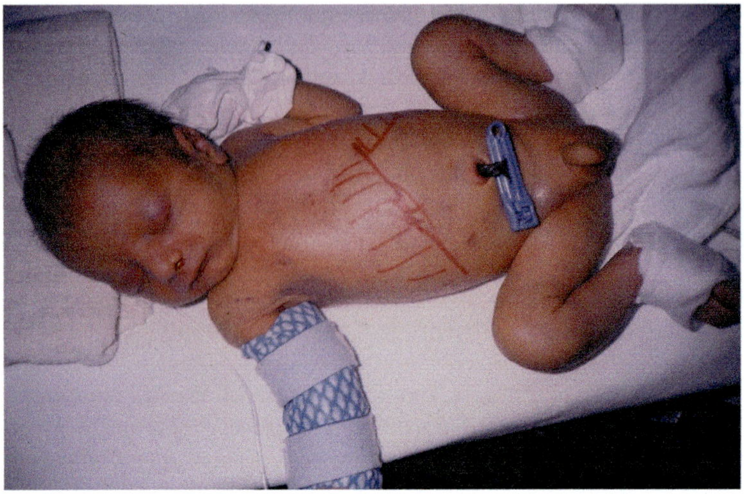

Fig. 5.1 Newborn with congenital CMV infection with hepatosplenomegaly (Photo: E. Rezanka)

early or late childhood. Therefore, the morbidity of CMV infection is devastating, due to its potential to cause cerebral palsy, cognitive impairment (50–80%), sensorineural hearing loss (30–60%), visual impairment (20–35%), neurodevelopmental behavioral, and neuromuscular disorders (30–60%; [9]).

5.5 Timing of Infection

Infections during early pregnancy more often result in more severe sequelae than infections later in pregnancy. About 10–20% of children with congenital CMV, asymptomatic or symptomatic in the neonatal period, will exhibit neurological damage when followed up [11]. Not all children with symptoms of congenital CMV infection in the neonatal period, though, may end up with sequelae: Up to one third of symptomatic neonates have been reported to have a normal outcome. In addition, not all children who are asymptomatic at birth will have a normal developmental outcome.

Infection early in pregnancy leads to intrauterine growth restriction with pronounced microcephaly and intracranial calcifications. Infection late in pregnancy more likely presents as acute visceral disease with hepatitis, pneumonitis, purpura, and severe thrombocytopenia [1]. Inflammatory infiltrate with focal necrosis is almost always present in CMV-infected fetal organs, and the severity of the inflammatory response correlates with organ damage in autoptic fetuses. However the damage in these organs is likely to be resolved by parenchymal regeneration.

CMV differs from other viruses with easy vertical transmission such as rubella as it can be transmitted to the fetus even if preconception maternal immunity is present. Its protective effect is demonstrated by a strongly decreasing incidence of vertical

Table 5.1 Symptomatic congenital CMV infection: common early symptoms

Organ system	Manifestation	%
	Symptoms at birth	10–20
	Asymptomatic at birth	80–90
	Mortality	7–30
	Growth retardation	50
	Prematurity	40
Liver	Hepatomegaly >3 cm	40–50
	Conjugated hyperbilirubinemia	50
	Elevated ALT or AST	40–50
Spleen	Splenomegaly	40–50
Platelets	Thrombocytopenia	40
	Intracranial hemorrhage	10
	Petechiae	40
Neurological system	Microcephaly <2 SD below mean	35–45
	Chorioretinitis	15–30
	Early sensorineural hearing loss	35
	Early seizures (onset <6 months)	15–25
	Abnormal EEG	50–67
	Abnormal brain MRI	87

transmission in which up to 40% of primary maternal infections, but less than 1% of recurrent infections, result in a congenitally infected child. It is generally accepted that symptoms of congenitally infected children are worse in case of primary rather than recurrent infection. However, severe symptoms due to congenital CMV infection after a recurrent maternal infection have been described also [12].

The clinical presentation is diversified as well as the range of sequelae and severity of adverse outcomes (Table 5.1): A large study [1] characterized clinical findings and adverse outcome in neonates with symptomatic congenital CMV infection and found the lowest common multiple to be hepatopathy, low platelets, and neurological findings.

The most commonly observed extra-neuronal symptoms at birth were intrauterine growth retardation (43%) and prematurity (29%) [1]. In detail, the extra-neurological manifestations were hepatosplenomegaly (50%), elevated transaminases (50%), thrombocytopenia (50%), conjugated hyperbilirubinemia (47%), and petechiae (45%).

Focal necroses, intrusion of inflammatory cell types, and inclusion-bearing cells were found in almost all placentas from symptomatic newborns. Finally, fetal death should be added to the list of possible sequelae resulting from maternal CMV infection.

5.6 Symptoms of the Central Nervous System in Detail

Among the primary clinical manifestations associated with congenital CMV infection, the most devastating are those involving the developing central nervous system, since in contrast to other end-organ injury, CNS injury is generally believed to be irreversible.

Central nervous infection results in focal encephalitis and periependymiditis. Once the acute phase is resolved, cicatrisation occurs via gliosis and calcification, which may be located at any place in the brain. Encephalitis involves cells of the white and gray matter as well as the choroid plexus. Viral inclusion-bearing cells are found in various neuronal and paraneuronal tissues and cells, e.g., neurons, ependyma, meninges, endothelium, choroid plexus, as well as in the inner ear (organ of Corti, cochlea), or in the eye. Brain damage, which seems to be the result of a combined effect of viral infection, inflammatory infiltration, and hypoxia due to severe placentitis, is less likely to be resolved because of the low regeneration ability of this organ.

Neuroradiological findings, associated with congenital CMV infection, include multifocal lesions predominantly involving deep parietal white matter, ventriculomegaly, intracranial calcifications, brain atrophy, and destructive encephalopathy, with or without gyral abnormalities, including lissencephaly, porencephaly, and schizencephaly. The presence of abnormalities in the anterior part of the temporal lobe increases the likelihood that CMV infection is present.

Brain abnormalities were mostly found in magnetic resonance imaging (75–89%) and head computed tomography scan (70%) with cerebral calcification in up to 60%. These methods in addition show abnormalities such as ventriculomegaly, white matter changes, polymicrogyria, cysts, structural abnormalities, and extensive encephalopathy. Other, very sensitive methods reveal abnormalities in brainstem auditory evoked responses (37%), visual evoked potentials (43%), and somatosensory evoked potentials (71%).

During early pregnancy, CMV is supposed to have teratogenic potential in the fetus, as CMV infections may result in migrational disturbances in the brain, as visualized by neuroimaging. Neocortical neurons migrate from their site of production in the extremely sensitive periventricular germinative zone toward the cortical plate between the 12th and 26th week of gestation. During this period, CMV may disturb the normal development of the brain and produce malformations [11]. A cohort of children with neurological disability and cerebral cortical malformations recognized by neuroimaging was tested in Sweden. The number of congenital CMV infections in children with cerebral cortical malformations was higher than expected with reference to the birth prevalence of congenital CMV infection, thus concluding that congenital CMV infection should be considered in children with cortical malformations of unknown origin [13]. Later in pregnancy, when the gross morphology of the brain is completed and myelination is occurring, white matter lesions without cerebral cortical malformations can be seen on magnetic resonance imaging (MRI), similar to those of inflammation [11, 14].

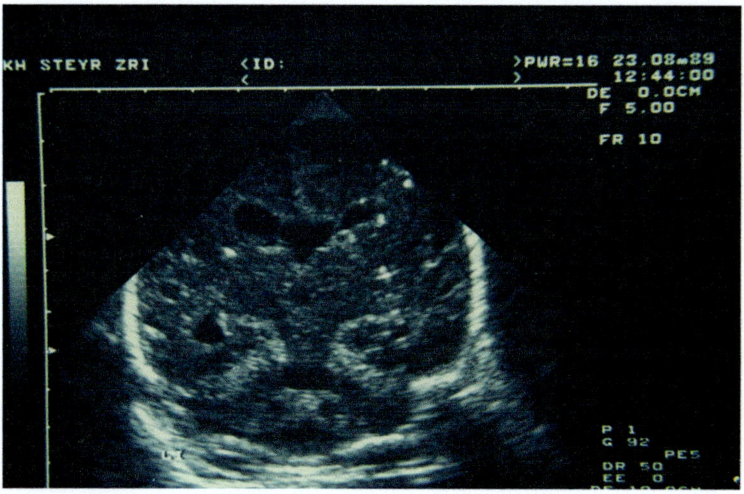

Fig. 5.2 Ultrasound image of the brain of a newborn with congenital CMV infection showing calcifications (Photo: E. Rezanka)

Pathologies in electroencephalographic methods are found in 40–60% of, including spikes, hypsarrhythmia. Abnormal results from cranial ultrasonograms are found in up to 70% of newborns with symptomatic CMV infection, showing calcifications (Fig. 5.2), usually periventricular or parenchymal in distribution, increased ventricular size, and cerebellar lesions. If these ultrasonograms are performed during the first week of life, they may be helpful for symptomatic children in predicting development of some neurological deficit in life. Typically, asymptomatic children do not show extensive calcifications or ventriculomegaly [15].

The disease causes a variety of disabilities, alone or in combination, such as delay in motor development (Fig. 5.3), mental retardation, learning disabilities, cerebral palsy, epilepsy, deafness or hearing impairment, and visual deficit or blindness. During the first year of life, severe damage including motor disability and severe mental retardation may be easy to diagnose, while mild mental retardation or learning disability without motor function deficit will become more obvious over time and can only be confirmed with neurodevelopmental assessment. Neurological symptoms due to CMV infection are relatively unique to congenital infection. In the CMV-infected adult, neurological complications are rare, except in cases of severe immunodeficiency (such as in advanced AIDS and organ transplant patients).

Factors associated with poor cognitive prognosis are microcephaly and abnormalities detected on computerized tomography or magnetic radiography imaging of the brain, as mentioned above. In contrast, children with normal findings on brain CT and a normal head circumference have been claimed to have a good cognitive outcome.

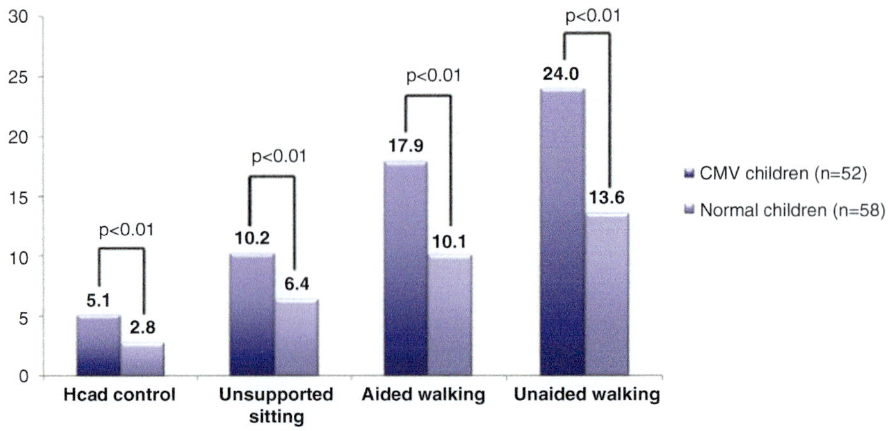

Fig. 5.3 Mean age (months for each postural–motor milestone in CMV-infected and normal children). From: X4. Audiovestibular consequences of congenital cytomegalovirus infection. Teissier N, Bernard S, Quesnel S, Van Den Abbeele T. Eur Ann Otorhinolaryngol Head Neck Dis. 2016 Dec;133(6):413–418

5.6.1 Microcephaly

Microcephaly usually is defined as the fronto-occipital head circumference below the fifth percentile. Pronounced forms of the disease often are characterized by circumferences 1–2 cm below the third percentile with more than two standard deviations below mean in up to 52%. In the past, when congenital CMV due to lack of sensitive diagnostic tools or clinical awareness was primarily detected via symptoms, microcephaly was the most prominent sign. However, in the series quoted above [1], only 37% of the symptomatic patients with connatal CMV were found microcephalic. The presence of microcephaly at birth was the most specific predictor of poor cognitive outcome in children with symptomatic congenital CMV infection, whereas children with normal findings on head CT and head circumference proportional to weight exhibited a good cognitive outcome [16]. The presence of intracellular calcifications is an additional negative prognostic predictor.

5.6.2 Ocular Defects

Main eye manifestation in CMV infection may lead to visual impairment and strabismus. These symptoms common in children with clinically apparent CMV infection can be caused by chorioretinitis, pigmentary retinitis, macular scarring, optic atrophy, and central cortical defects. The reported incidence of chorioretinitis in symptomatic neonates varies from 15 to 30%. Visual impairment in infants without clinical signs in the newborn period is unusual [11]. Microphthalmus, cataracts, retinal necrosis and calcification, anterior chamber, and optic disk malformation have also been described in association with generalized infection but are far less common [17]. On the base of appearance, ocular lesions, caused by CMV, cannot be distinguished from those caused by *Toxoplasma gondii*; however, postnatal progression of the latter is rather uncommon.

5.6.3 Hearing Loss

Congenital CMV infection is the most important single cause of sensorineural hearing loss or deafness during childhood. Because sensorineural hearing loss is the most common sequela of connatal CMV infection, it is a major contributor to disease burden. A meta-analysis showed that with a prevalence of connatal CMV in developed countries of 0.58% (95% confidence interval, 0.41–0.79), 12.6% (95% confidence interval, 10.2–16.5) will experience hearing loss: One out of three symptomatic children and one out of ten asymptomatic children. Among symptomatic children, the majority have bilateral loss; among asymptomatic children, unilateral loss predominates. In both groups the hearing loss is mainly severe to profound [18].

The hearing loss may occur late onset during the first 6 years of life in children with both symptomatic and asymptomatic infection in the neonatal period [11, 19]. - CMV-induced hearing loss is believed to be caused by virus-induced labyrinthitis. Identified risk factors for sensorineural hearing loss in connatal CMV infection comprise a symptomatic infection at birth (OR = 9.3), a viral load >5000 plaque-forming units (PFU) in urine, and 10,000 copies/ml in blood, delayed intrauterine growth, indicating both fetal and placental infection. In contrast, hepatosplenomegaly, hepatitis, intracerebral calcification, and thrombopenia do not seem to be risk factors (reviewed in [20]). Inner ear histology from congenitally infected infants shows damage to structures including the vestibular endolymphatic system and the vestibular organs and collapse of the saccular membrane [15]. Hearing loss from congenital CMV infection can be either unilateral or bilateral and varies from mild to profound in terms of degree [17]. Reportedly, approximately half of hearing losses due to congenital CMV infection are late onset or progressive and, therefore, cannot be detected at birth through newborn hearing screening [21]. Congenital CMV infection following primary maternal infection during the first trimester of pregnancy is more likely to lead to central nervous system sequelae than fetal infection due to maternal infection later in pregnancy, showed in a large prospective study: Sensorineural hearing loss was found in 24% of children in the first trimester group, compared with only in the later infection group. Considering any CNS sequela (hearing loss, mental retardation, cerebral palsy, seizures, chorioretinitis), 32% first trimester cases were affected compared with 15% in the later infection group. None of the latter group had more than one sequela, compared with 12% of the first trimester group

5.6.4 Mental and Psychomotor Retardation

With symptomatic congenital CMV infection survived, the likelihood of survival with normal intellect is low. Psychomotor retardation is mostly combined with microcephaly and occurs in nearly 70% of the patients. In a large study [16], almost one third of children with symptomatic congenital CMV infection had a normal cognitive outcome. The presence of microcephaly at birth, when carefully assessed, by adjusting for gestational age and weight, was the most specific predictor of poor cognitive outcome in children with symptomatic congenital CMV infection. Psychomotor retardation in various forms as tetra and diplegia is described.

5.6.5 Seizures

Infants with congenital CMV infections can demonstrate very intense and drug-resistant forms of epilepsy. Seizures may be one of the first clinical symptoms and signs of CMV infection, starting in the neonatal period or later during the first year of life, e.g., generalized tonic-clonic seizures, polymorphic seizures, infantile spasms, or West syndrome in childhood. This relationship has been known for almost 40 years. Epileptic spasms usually begin between the third and the sixth month of life. The diagnosis of West syndrome is made by the existence of infantile spasm; flexor postures of sudden onset between the age of 3 and 7 months, by an interictal EEG pattern termed hypsarrhythmia; and mental retardation. This severe epilepsy syndrome is an age-dependent expression of a damaged brain.

Seizures can also lead to regression in psychomotor development. The vast majority of patients may require polytherapy in order to become seizure-free. In patients with severe brain damage in neuroimaging examinations and/or hypsarrhythmia in the electroencephalography, results of combined antiviral and antiepileptic therapy were generally poor [22], and only early antiviral and antiepileptic therapy could result in the long-term cessation of seizures.

5.7 Unspecific Symptoms in Detail

5.7.1 Temperature Instability

In up to 10%, as shown in prospective studies, an acute, progressive form of disease is present. As a symptom of systemic involvement, newborns may present with high fever, which, for conditions of preterms or term newborns, reaches unusual peak values of up to 39.5°C. Therefore, if fever is the leading symptom, possibly accompanied by rash, or grayish skin color, pallor, or petechia, congenital CMV infection clinically may present as an early onset sepsis. In fulminant courses, as this holds true for neonatal sepsis too, temperature instability (>2°C), or even hypothermia (<36.5°C), may be present in severely ill patients.

5.7.2 Perfusion and Rash

Newborns may have a poor skin perfusion with a capillary refill of more than 2–3 s, arterial hypotension with a mean arterial blood pressure below gestational age, and to a lesser extent tachycardia with a heart rate of more than 160 beats per minute. General but unspecific symptoms are muscular hypotonia, irritability, hyperexcitability, neck stiffness, lethargy, hyper- or hypoglycemia, gastric residues or vomiting, and abdominal distension. The skin may present with localized macular papules within the face, a purpuric rash, resembling systemic rubella infection, or "blueberry muffin" spots, resembling leukemic or syphilitic efflorescences.

5.7.3 Lung

The pulmonary reaction tends to be mild and often clinically inapparent but involves inflammation of alveolar cells with the signs of pneumonitis. Thus, a common symptom is moderate tachypnea with 60–80 respirations per minute at rest, accompanied by dyspnea with grunting, nasal flaring, and costal retractions, which easily can be detected but, in the coincidence of prematurity, hypotrophy, or sectio caesarea, may be misdiagnosed as transitionary wet lung or respiratory distress syndrome. In preterm infants, apnea and bradycardia may appear progressively, leading to respiratory insufficiency and secondary intubation and ventilation.

5.7.4 Liver

Hepatomegaly is one of the most common clinical signs for congenital CMV infection in the neonate, resulting from a mild and often transient hepatitis. Liver enzymes, in particular transaminases, are moderately elevated, and liver function tests may be abnormal; however, in most cases not to the extent, coagulation is severely altered, so that substitution with fresh frozen plasma rarely has to occur. In the majority of patients, the liver edge is smooth and non-tender and usually measures 4–9 cm below the right costal margin, but a firm, palpable and in size within days increasing organ as well has been described.

5.7.5 Jaundice

This symptom occurs chameleon-like, inconstantly, and in various forms: The most form of hyperbilirubinemia in the active disease is an icterus praecox et gravis either already present at birth or occurring rapidly soon after with an elevation of the unconjugated and conjugated fraction of bilirubin. The latter component usually increases within the course of time, leading to a distribution of up to 60% of the total bilirubin. Since hyperbilirubinemia is caused by hepatic inflammation, it may develop into an icterus prolongatus, present within the first weeks of life and fluctuating within time. Other newborns present with only transient and mild jaundice, vanishing within days or weeks.

5.7.6 Spleen

Although splenomegaly is a common symptom, sometimes occurring as the only clinical abnormality, present in a routine examination and in up to 85% of all symptomatic congenital infections, it is not diagnosed too easily, since the enlargement reaches up to 15 cm below the costal margin and consists of a soft swelling; therefore it may be failed to touch. In the course of disease, splenomegaly may be progressive over days.

5.7.7 Platelet System

CMV infection negatively affects megakarycytosis in the bone marrow. In addition to it, platelets are eliminated via sequestration in the enlarged organs of the liver and spleen. The most common hematologic abnormalities consist of anemia and thrombocytopenia. The latter mostly is mild (i.e., >50,000/mm^3), asymptomatic, and transient, so at a large majority of patients, thrombocytopenia resolves within 2 weeks, and there is no need for platelet transfusions. If thrombocytopenia persists with bleeding tendencies and/or platelet counts are below 20,000/mm^3, repeated platelet transfusions especially in premature infants are required. Petechiae, often appearing disseminated or localized in regions of mechanical alteration within a few hours after birth, may be transient and vanish after several days, in some cases, however, persist for weeks. It is remarkable that petechial rashes are not necessarily combined with low platelet counts and that mechanical alteration may provoke the appearance of petechiae also later in the course of disease.

5.7.8 Anemia

CMV-induced hemolysis leads to chronic anemia in which the exact pathomechanisms are not fully understood. Again, red blood cell trapping via hypersplenismus and sequestration are involved in these processes. As a consequence, extramedullary hematopoiesis often occurs, resulting in erythroblastemia. Anemia rarely is life-threatening and resolves within the first 12–18 months of life.

5.7.9 Gastrointestinal Tract

Intestinal CMV-infected cells in infants have prevalently been associated with neonatal necrotizing enterocolitis, a most serious complication, mainly affecting preterm neonates. However, gastrointestinal involvement is usually not included in

Table 5.2 Symptomatic congenital CMV infection: neurological deficits >2 years of age (modified: Kylat et al. [1])

Organ	Manifestation	%
	Deaths	5–10
Ear	Late hearing loss (moderate + severe)	30–65
Eye	Visual loss/severe impairment	10–20
Brain	Cognitive defects	50–70
	Motor deficit (mild to severe)	60–80
	Developmental delay	60–80
	Speech delay	80
	Bedridden or wheelchair bound	10–20

the clinical spectrum of congenital CMV infections [9], whereas, in contrast, in adults CMV-associated infection in the gastrointestinal tract is not uncommon. Over the last years, several case reports of CMV-associated NEC in infants have been reported. None of the reports though clearly stated whether CMV was directly responsible for the NEC or a manifestation of superinfection. Single case reports were described with gastrointestinal involvement, developing a colonic stricture and manifesting a clinical picture simulating Hirschsprung's disease. Intestinal lesions, identified as localized segmental CMV infection of the colon, dominated the histopathological findings [23].

5.8 Asymptomatic Infection

Asymptomatic infection, as indicated in the previous section, affects the highest proportion of infants with congenital CMV infection. Long-term problems related to infected children's growth and early clinical use of antiviral drugs are still unclear. Studies indicate that asymptomatic congenital CMV infection, most importantly, has an impact on infant hearing loss (Table 5.2), since 10–15% of them are equally at risk for sensorineural sequelae, like 20–30% of all the infected children. As many as 5% of children with congenital CMV infection develop moderate to profound bilateral hearing loss by 6 years of age, and up to 15% of children develop any type. Therefore it is important that a time prolonged and closer follow-up of infected children should be until 6 years of age. This should lead to an early intervention and better management and eventually even control the long-term sequelae [24].

5.9 Differential Diagnosis

Common differential diagnoses are other congenital infections such as toxoplasmosis, rubella, herpes simplex, acquired immune deficiency syndrome, and syphilis. Such distinction is possible, both clinically and serologically.

Congenital toxoplasmosis is an embryofoetopathy with mostly normal development, but up to 4% of the patients die or have evidence of permanent neurological damage or bilateral visual impairment during the first years of age. In contrast to

CMV infection, toxoplasmosis is more likely to be associated with an isolated chorioretinitis, microphthalmia, hydrocephalus, and scattered cerebral calcifications. Petechial and purpuric eruptions, which are common in symptomatic congenital CMV infections, are rare in congenital toxoplasmosis; the latter often presents with a maculopapular rash.

Rubella causes congenital malformations realizing the Gregg's tripod: ocular lesions, mainly cataracts, congenital heart disease with cardiac lesions (ventricular septal defects, pulmonary stenosis, combined defects), and neurological manifestations characterized by sensorineural deafness. According to some authors, "salt and pepper" chorioretinitis, involving the periphery and the posterior pole of the retina, is more frequently found in congenital rubella [25]; intracerebral calcification is missing.

Grouped skin vesicles or scarring present at birth suggests congenital herpes simplex infection, whereas stigmata mainly involving skin and extremities may point to congenital varicella zoster infection with its characteristic cutaneous lesion known as cicatrix, a zigzag scarring often in the dermatomal distribution.

Rhinitis and radiological evidence of osteochondritis and epiphysitis favor the diagnosis of congenital syphilis. A much more common differential diagnosis includes bacterial sepsis and erythroblastosis fetalis. Metabolic disorders such as galactosemia and tyrosinemia may as well be considered, especially if hypoglycemia or acidosis is present.

References

1. Kylat RI, Kelly EN, Ford-Jones EL (2005) Clinical findings and adverse outcome in neonates with symptomatic congenital cytomegalovirus (SCCMV) infection. Eur J Pediatr 165:773–778
2. Cannon MJ, Davis FK (2005) Washing our hands of the congenital cytomegalovirus disease epidemic. BMC Public Health 5:70
3. Ludwig A, Hengel H (2009) Epidemiological impact and disease burden of congenital cytomegalovirus infection in Europe. Euro Surveill 14:1
4. Lanzieri TM, Dollard SC, Bialek SR et al (2014) Systematic review of the birth prevalence of congenital cytomegalovirus infection in developing countries. Int J Infect Dis 22:44–48
5. Emery VC, Lazzarotto T (2017) Cytomegalovirus in pregnancy and the neonate. F1000Res 6:138. https://doi.org/10.12688/f1000research.10276.1
6. Boppana SB, Fowler KB, Britt WJ, Stagno S, Pass RF (1999) Symptomatic congenital cytomegalovirus infection in infants born to mothers with preexisting immunity to cytomegalovirus. Pediatrics 104:55–60
7. Andriesse GI, Weersink AJ, de Boer J (2006) Visual impairment and deafness in young children: consider the diagnosis of congenital infection with cytomegalovirus, even years after birth. Arch Ophthalmol 124:743
8. Boppana SB, Fowler KB, Pass RF, Rivera LB, Bradford RD, Lakeman FD, Britt WJ (2005) Congenital cytomegalovirus infection: association between virus burden in infancy and hearing loss. J Pediatr 146:817–823
9. Stagno S, Britt B (2006) Cytomegalovirus. In: Remington JS, Klein JO, Wilson CB, Baker CJ (eds) Infectious diseases of the fetus and newborn infant, 6th edn. Elsevier Saunders, Philadelphia, pp 740–781
10. Leung AK, Sauve RS, Davies HD (2003) Congenital cytomegalovirus infection. J Natl Med Assoc 95:213–218

11. Malm G, Engman ML (2007) Congenital cytomegalovirus infections. Semin Fetal Neonatal Med 12:154–159
12. Gaytant MA, Rours GI, Steegers EA, Galama JM, Semmekrot BA (2003) Congenital cytomegalovirus infection after recurrent infection: case reports and review of the literature. Eur J Pediatr 162:248–253
13. Engman ML, Lewensohn-Fuchs I, Mosskin M, Malm G (2010) Congenital cytomegalovirus infection: the impact of cerebral cortical malformations. Acta Paediatr 99:1344–1349
14. Jones CA (2003) Congenital cytomegalovirus infection. Curr Prob Pediatr Adolesc Health Care 33:100
15. Cheeran MC, Lokensgard JR, Schleiss MR (2009) Neuropathogenesis of congenital cytomegalovirus infection: disease mechanisms and prospects for intervention. Clin Microbiol Rev 22:99–126
16. Noyola DE, The Houston Congenital CMV Longitudinal Study Group (2001) Early predictors of neurodevelopmental outcome in symptomatic congenital cytomegalovirus infection. J Pediatr 138:325–331
17. Pass RF, Fowler KB, Boppana SB, Britt WJ, Stagno S (2006) Congenital cytomegalovirus infection following first trimester maternal infection: symptoms at birth and outcome. J Clin Virol 53:216–220
18. Goderis J, De Leenheer E, Smets K, Van Hoecke H, Keymeulen A, Dhooge I (2014) Hearing loss and congenital CMV infection: a systematic review. Pediatrics 134(5):972–982
19. Dahle AJ, Fowler KB, Wright JD, Boppana SB, Britt WJ, Pass RFI (2000) Longitudinal investigation of hearing disorders in children with congenital cytomegalovirus. J Am Acad Audiol 11:283–290
20. Teissier N, Bernard S, Quesnel S, Van Den Abbeele T (2016) Audiovestibular consequences of congenital cytomegalovirus infection. Eur Ann Otorhinolaryngol Head Neck Dis 133(6): 413–418
21. Fowler KB, Dahle AJ, Boppana SB, Pass RF (1999) Newborn hearing screening: will children with hearing loss caused by congenital cytomegalovirus infection be missed? J Pediatr 135:60–64
22. Dunin-Wasowicz D, Kasprzyk-Obara J, Jurkiewicz E, Kapusta M, Milewska-Bobula B (2007) Infantile spasms and cytomegalovirus infection: antiviral and antiepileptic treatment. Dev Med Child Neurol 49:684–692
23. Ekema G, Pedersini P, Milianti S, Ubertazzi M, Minoli D, Manciana A (2006) Colonic stricture mimicking Hirschsprung's disease: a localized cytomegalovirus infection. J Pediatr Surg 41: 850–852
24. Lombardi G, Garofoli F, Stronati M (2010) Congenital cytomegalovirus infection: treatment, sequelae and follow-up. J Matern Fetal Neonatal Med 23(Suppl 3):45–48
25. Eballe AO, Ellong A, Zoua ME, Bella LA, Ngeufack S, Kouam JM, Melong J (2010) Cerebral and ocular congenital toxoplasmosis complicated by West syndrome. Clin Ophthalmol 4:861–864

6 Prevention and Therapy: More than Trial and Error

Gabriele Halwachs-Baumann

Primum non nocere
(First, do no harm)

Scribonius Largus, 50 AD

Given the importance of congenital CMV as a potentially preventable cause of disability in children, it is logical to consider it for potential inclusion in public health newborn screening [1]. This statement is in polar opposite to an opinion published 2 years before, concluding that no screening program for congenital cytomegalovirus infection is justified [2]. These two examples stand for two groups of scientists, the one being optimistic seeing a benefit in promoting CMV awareness in the community and the other being afraid to open Pandora's box [1–4]. It is written: "For in much wisdom is much grief: and he that increases the knowledge increases the sorrow" (Ecclesiastes 1:18). But it is also written: "The simple believes everything, but the prudent looks where he is going." (Proverbs 14:15). In the absence of proven therapeutic options, prevention of CMV infection in women of reproductive age is an important strategy to reduce the rate of congenital CMV infection. And the easiest way to prevent congenital cytomegalovirus is the teaching and implementation of hygiene interventions [4]. We now know the risk factors for congenital cytomegalovirus infection. Caring for preschool children is one of them [5–7]. The problem is the lack of knowledge and awareness of congenital cytomegalovirus among women. Only 13–22% of women had heard of congenital CMV (and only 7% of men), compared to 98% who had heard of HIV/AIDS [8, 9]. Thereby seroconversion rates consistently decrease as cytomegalovirus education and

G. Halwachs-Baumann (✉)
Department of Laboratory Medicine, Regional Hospital Steyr, Steyr, Austria
e-mail: gabriele.baumann@gespag.at

G. Halwachs-Baumann (ed.), *Congenital Cytomegalovirus Infection*,
https://doi.org/10.1007/978-3-319-98770-5_6

support increases [10, 11]. Hygienic practices to reduce risk of CMV infection for women who are pregnant or planning to become pregnant are simple [8]:

1. Thoroughly wash hands with soap and warm water after activities such as:
   Diaper changes.
   Feeding or bathing child.
   Wiping child's runny nose or drool.
   Handling child's toys.
2. Do not share cups, plates, utensils, toothbrushes, or food.
3. Do not kiss on or near the mouth.
4. Do not share towels or washcloths.
5. Clean toys, countertops, and other surfaces that come in contact with urine or saliva.

As mentioned above studies of hygiene education have shown that increasing the awareness in seronegative pregnant women for the risk of CMV transfer from their firstborn or their partners can decrease seroconversion dramatically [12]. So in an Italian study, 1.2% seroconverted in the intervention group compared to 7.6% in the comparison group [13]. The reduction of CMV infection by educating women was even more impressive comparing pregnant mothers with nonpregnant women. In the first group, only 3% CMV infections were observed, whereas in the second group, 42% CMV infections have been seen [6, 14]. The effectiveness of handwashing to remove viable CMV was proven in an artificial setting using different cleansing agents. Even using just normal water led to a complete erase of viable virus [15].

Besides these educating behavioral changes, therapy with antivirals, prevention and/or therapy by administering CMV-specific hyperimmunoglobulin, and active immunization/vaccination are discussed strategies.

6.1 Antivirals

Several CMV inhibitors can be used to treat CMV disease in allograft recipients and patients with AIDS. Ganciclovir is currently the gold standard for the treatment of CMV diseases [16, 17]. This drug consists of a guanine linked to an acyclic sugar-like molecule which lacks the equivalent of the $2'CH_2$ moiety. Ganciclovir undergoes a first step of phosphorylation by the CMV UL97 protein kinase and is then converted by cellular kinases to the triphosphate form. This chemical form interacts with the viral polymerase and inhibits DNA synthesis by competing with the natural nucleoside. Ganciclovir is currently available as an intravenous formulation [17].

Valganciclovir is a prodrug of ganciclovir that has an oral bioavailability of around 60% [11, 12]. Beside these two drugs, foscarnet and cidofovir are licensed for the systemic treatment of CMV infection. Beside these pharmaceuticals, acyclovir and its prodrug valacyclovir were described to be effective against CMV, albeit in a higher dosage than used for the treatment of herpes simplex infection or chicken pox [18], due to the less efficient phosphorylation of acyclovir by UL97 [19]. These observations were mainly made in transplant recipients. Nevertheless, beside some case reports for foscarnet [20], ganciclovir and valganciclovir are the only two medications that have been employed in the treatment of congenital CMV infection to date [21].

Pharmacokinetic studies in infants and neonates evaluating oral valganciclovir at a dose of 16 mg/kg every 12 h and intravenous ganciclovir at a dose of 6 mg/kg every 12 h have shown similar areas under the plasma concentration-time curve for both drugs [22–25]. So both medications seem to be effective in the treatment of congenital cytomegalovirus disease.

Some studies exist using valacyclovir for the treatment of pregnant women. This drug was chosen, since there are less side effects of valacyclovir compared to ganciclovir or this prodrug. The hesitative use of ganciclovir/valganciclovir in pregnant women is a consequence of the teratogenic and hematopoietic adverse effects of these substances [26].

6.1.1 Treatment of Pregnant Women

Antiviral therapy of infected mothers has reduced the transmission of HIV dramatically [16, 27]. For ganciclovir experiments on the perfused placenta have shown that this nucleoside analogue can cross the placenta quite well [27]. Nevertheless, the implications of fetal risk are an important aspect of drug treatment for pregnant women. There exist only a few studies using antivirals to treat CMV infection during pregnancy. In the study of Jacquemard et al. [26], valacyclovir was offered to 20 women with 21 symptomatic CMV-positive fetuses. Therapeutic concentrations were achieved in maternal and fetal bloods. The viral load in the fetal blood decreased significantly after 1–12 weeks of treatment. For methodological reasons, it was not possible to assess whether treatment with valacyclovir reduced the severity of disease by comparison with an untreated group [26]. Another study included 41 pregnant women and their 43 fetuses [28]. As it was shown in the abovementioned study, valacyclovir reduced the viral load in the blood of the fetus. Comparison of results of this trial with those of an historical cohort indicates that valacyclovir increased the proportion of asymptomatic neonates, from 43% without treatment to 82% with treatment. To prove the efficacy of this treatment, a prospective randomized controlled trial is still lacking.

Reports on treatment of pregnant women with ganciclovir/valganciclovir are even less. Only a few case reports describe the administration of these antivirals or this indication. As for acyclovir/valacyclovir, viral load was reduced in the blood of the fetus/newborn [29]. Since there is no established way to predict postnatal outcome in fetal CMV infection, no conclusion on efficacy of this therapy on prevention of symptoms can be made. As evidence on safety is lacking, ganciclovir/valganciclovir administration during pregnancy in the setting of fetal CMV infection is not recommended in a recently published consensus statement [30].

6.1.2 Treatment of Neonates

Since the early 1990s, case reports and studies with small numbers of patients were published [31–34]. Later on controlled trials were published, using different therapeutic regimen [34–38] (Table 6.1). In all trials an improvement or stabilization was seen at least concerning hearing. Shedding of CMV in urine was also temporarily reduced during treatment [35, 38, 40]. Case reports demonstrated the beneficial effect of antiviral treatment on chorioretinitis [41, 42].

Due to a more feasible mode of administration, valganciclovir monotherapy [24, 25, 43] or followed after ganciclovir therapy [44] was assessed, leading to comparable results to the ganciclovir trials. Major side effects observed in these infants treated with antivirals were thrombocytopenia and neutropenia and bacterial infection of the catheter in those children with long time i.v. ganciclovir treatment. Based on the to-date published data 2010, an evidence-based approach on the management of congenital cytomegalovirus infection was published [45]. The authors' recommendation grade B for the treatment of neonates with congenital CMV infection says that either 6 mg/kg ganciclovir i.v. twice a week or 15 mg/kg oral valganciclovir twice a day can be used. Treatment should not exceed 6 weeks. Monitoring of the full blood count, liver function tests, creatinine, urea, and electrolytes should be done three times weekly. As indications for suspension, an absolute neutrophil count <500 cells/µl and/or platelet count <25,000 cells/µl was recommended [45]. In the 2017 published consensus recommendations, valganciclovir treatment at a dosage of 16 mg/kg/dose given twice daily for 6 months

Table 6.1 Dosage and duration of ganciclovir treatment

		Dosage	Duration
Nigro et al. [34]	Group 1	5 mg/kg twice daily	2 weeks
	Group 2	7.5 mg/kg twice daily thereafter 10 mg/kg three times a week	2 weeks 3 months
Halwachs-Baumann et al. [36]		10 mg/kg twice daily	3 weeks
Whitley et al. [35]	Group 1	8 mg/kg twice daily	6 weeks
		12 mg/kg twice daily	6 weeks
Michaels et al. [37] and Jacquemard et al. [26]		10 mg/kg/day thereafter 5 mg/kg/day Subsequent orally ganciclovir 550 mg/m^2/dose three times a day	2–4 weeks Median 12 months (5.5–18 months) Median 10 months (6 months–3 years)
Kimberlin et al. [38]		Ganciclovir 6 mg/kg/dose given every 12 h i.v.	6 weeks
Kimberlin et al. [24]		Valganciclovir 16 mg/kg/dose twice daily orally	6 weeks
Kimberlin et al. [39]		Valganciclovir 16 mg/kg/dose twice daily orally	6 months

is recommended for congenitally infected neonates with moderately to severely symptomatic disease [30, 39].

There is still debate on the selection of neonates with congenital cytomegalovirus infection for antiviral therapy [46–50]. Consent exists on the therapeutic intervention if the neonate has symptoms at birth. Infants with virologically confirmed congenital CMV should undergo complete physical examination and focused laboratory and imaging evaluation to determine the extent of disease [49, 50]. There is no debate to treat neonates with life-threatening infections, those with central nervous system involvement, and those with abnormal laboratory findings (e.g., thrombocytopenia) and petechiae (due to the possible affection of their long-term neurodevelopmental outcome). No consent exists on antiviral therapy of asymptomatic newborns, although it is known that these children can develop permanent neurologic sequelae [51, 52]. Thus, asymptomatic congenital CMV infection is a leading cause of sensorineural hearing loss in young children. Long-time follow-up of asymptomatic congenitally CMV-infected newborns has shown that i.v. ganciclovir therapy has a beneficial effect on the hearing development. None of the children, diagnosed having asymptomatic congenital CMV infection in the first week after birth, nevertheless treated with ganciclovir, and re-examined at the age of 4–11 years, showed an abnormal sensorineural hearing status. Whereas, 2/8 asymptomatic, nontreated children showed sensorineural hearing loss at the age of 8 and 10 years, respectively [53]. Perhaps these preliminary data lead to a new thinking on therapeutic options in congenitally CMV-infected children asymptomatic at birth. At present for asymptomatic congenitally CMV-infected children, only hearing is tested every 6 months for 3 years, and then yearly for at least an additional 1–2 year is recommended. Any defects should be identified and addressed with appropriate nonpharmacologic interventions [54].

Beside potential toxicities [22], the major limitation of antiviral therapy for congenital CMV infection is the fact that much of the CNS damage occurs in utero, prior to the ability of recognition. So prevention of an intrauterine infection of the child may offer a better solution [55].

6.2 Passive Immunization

Immunoglobulin preparations were first made available for therapeutic use in the 1950s. The problems and side effects with the initial preparations have been resolved long ago [56, 57]. Nowadays, regarding safety, intravenous immunoglobulins are the most purified among the blood derivatives, including albumin, and are the only derivatives which can be pasteurized. For intravenous immunoglobulins, in over 17 years of use, no case of viral transmission has been reported [58].

The administration of i.v. immunoglobulin preparations is now widely used for prevention and treatment of bacterial as well as viral infections [59]. In bacterial disease, antibodies neutralize toxins, facilitate opsonization, and, with complement, promote bacteriolysis; in viral disease, antibodies block viral entry into uninfected cells, promote antibody-directed cell-mediated cytotoxicity by natural killer cells, and neutralize virus alone or with the participation of complement [59]. The use of hyperimmunoglobulin in the prevention and control of hepatitis A and B virus is well established and its positive effect well proven in the adult and in the neonate [59–63]. Also in other diseases, the beneficial effect is documented [64–66]. Concerning passive immunization of the mother, the gestational age-dependent transfer via the placenta has to be considered. Although IgG and IgA are potentially available to the embryo as early as the 6th week of gestation, active transport across the placenta is increasing with advancing gestation [67].

Preconceptional CMV immunity is known to have a protective effect against CMV infection following intense exposure to the virus in the secretions of young children attending group day care [68]. This preconceptional immunity must have high titers of neutralizing antibodies. The mechanism of passive immunization works by imitating a seropositive status, as it is produced by a CMV wild-type infection. The currently available immunoglobulin preparations have anti-gB titers of 1/400,000. This is approximately two- to fourfold higher than that observed among individuals naturally seropositive for CMV. The commercially available hyperimmune globulin preparations Cytogam (in the USA available CMV hyperimmune globulin) and Cytotect (in Europe available CMV hyperimmune globulin) also contain very high titers of antibodies that block viral entry into endothelial and epithelial cells [58, 69].

The mode of action of CMV-specific hyperimmune globulin is very complex and yet not fully understood. Animal models have shown the protective effect of CMV-specific antibodies. In the brains of murine CMV-infected newborn mice treated with CMV-specific immune serum, the titer of infectious virus was reduced below detection limit, whereas in the brains of mice receiving control (nonimmune) serum, significant amounts of virus were recovered. Moreover, histopathological and immunohistological analyses revealed significantly less CNS inflammation in mice treated with CMV immune serum. Recipients of control serum or irrelevant antibodies had more viral foci, marked mononuclear cell infiltrates, and prominent glial nodules in their brains [70]. This protective effect of passive immunization on the developing CNS might explain observations of resolution of fetal abnormalities due to intrauterine CMV infection [71–75]. Despite this, there are several plausible mechanisms for the therapeutic efficacy of passive immunization: immunomodulatory effects, reduction of maternal viremia and viral load, and decreased placental inflammation resulting in increased blood flow with enhanced fetal nutrition, oxygenation, and survival [58]. Most notably the role of the placenta seems to be important in the context of congenital CMV infection. Placentas of women with primary CMV infection who have a fetus or newborn with CMV disease are significantly thicker than those of women with primary CMV infection who don't have a diseased fetus or newborn. The receipt of hyperimmune globulin is associated with statistically significant reduction in placental thickness [76]. This publication depicts the crucial role of the placenta in the context of congenital CMV infection. Much of the injury that CMV produces in the newborn may be caused by placental insufficiency and injury and not by viral infection of the fetus, per se. Thus, one of the beneficial effects of hyperimmune globulin may be mediated through improved placental health [77].

One of the most exiting works concerning prevention and treatment of congenital CMV infection was the 2005 published paper of Nigro et al. [75]. It provoked an intense and emotional debate in the scientific community [78–85]. This paper described the prevention and treatment of congenital CMV infection by administering CMV-specific hyperimmune globulin to pregnant women. It was a multicenter prospective cohort study including 181 pregnant women with confirmed primary CMV infection. The therapy group comprised women whose amniotic fluid contained either CMV or CMV DNA. These women were offered with intravenous hyperimmune globulin at a dose of 200 U/kg of maternal weight. Additional intravenous doses and intra-umbilical cord or intra-amniotic doses (400 U/kg of fetal weight) were used only in the event of ultrasonographic evidence of persistent fetal involvement. The prevention group comprised women who had not undergone amniocentesis before or at enrolment. Reasons for not undergoing amniocentesis were a primary infection within 6 weeks before enrolment and a pregnancy of less than 20 week's gestation or women declining to undergo the procedure. All women were offered intravenous hyperimmune globulin at a dose of 100 U/kg every month until delivery.

From 31 women included in the therapy group who received hyperimmune globulin, only 1 delivered an infant with CMV disease, whereas 7 of 14 women who did not receive hyperimmune globulin had affected infants. In the prevention group, 37 women received hyperimmune globulin, 6 of whom had infants with congenital CMV infection, as compared with 19 of 47 women who did not receive hyperimmune globulin. So, the authors concluded that CMV-specific hyperimmune globulin reduces the severity of symptoms in congenitally CMV-infected newborns and reduces the risk of CMV transmission from mother to child [75]. No adverse events were associated with hyperimmune globulin infusions.

In contrast to these results in a follow-up study, the difference of the rate of congenital CMV-infected newborns between hyperimmune globulin-treated group and placebo-treated group (30% vs. 44%) was not statistically significant, whereas the number of obstetrical adverse events was higher in the hyperimmune globulin group (13% vs. 2%) [86]. Subsequent studies did not confirm the observation of side effects. Contrariwise they described hyperimmunoglobulin administration during pregnancy as safe and not associated with prematurity or decreased birth weight [87–89]. Since these clinical studies do not provide information on the CMV infection status of the fetus prior to the start of hyperimmunoglobulin administration, it cannot be said whether this treatment has been therapeutic or prophylactic in the one or the other case [90].

Beside case reports there exist only limited data on the therapeutic use of hyperimmunoglobulin during pregnancy. In 2012 Visentin et al. [91] published data on hyperimmunoglobulin treatment in 31 women compared to 36 women with no treatment. CMV DNA was identified in the amniotic fluid of all fetuses. At the 1-year evaluation, 4/31 infants of treated women showed a poor outcome in contrast to 16/37 infants of nontreated women.

To elucidate the effect of CMV hyperimmunoglobulin administration on the rate and severity of congenital CMV infection (prophylactic or therapeutic use), phase III studies are on the way. As now presumed completion date will be at the end of 2018. Nevertheless, until results of controlled trials are available, off-label use of CMV-specific hyperimmune globulin seems to be justified, since the maxim *primum non nocere* (first, do no harm) is fulfilled, one of the principal precepts of medical ethics, first framed by Scribonius Largus, physician at the court of Emperor Tiberius Claudius (50 AD).

6.3 Active Immunization (Vaccination)

First of all, there is no licensed CMV vaccine currently available, although the search for an effective vaccine still lasts for a long time [92–98]. There exist several approaches for the development of a CMV vaccine: (1) purified recombinant gB subunit vaccines, (2) enveloped virus-like particles (eVLP) vaccines, (3) vectored CMV vaccines, (4) nucleic acid-based CMV vaccines, (5) live attenuated and "disc" vaccines, and (6) peptide vaccines [99–103] (Table 6.2). Nevertheless, the development of an effective vaccine turned out to be difficult due to the complex virus host interaction. As mentioned in Chap. 2, there exist distinct pathways for CMV entry into fibroblasts (receptor-mediated fusion infection pathway) and into endothelial, epithelial, and dendritic cells (endosomal infection pathway) [104]. These findings explain why Towne and gB vaccines, effective in neutralizing fibroblast infection, fail to inhibit infection of epithelial cells equally to natural infection, since the majority of the neutralizing activity of convalescent human sera from CMV-seropositive individuals targets the endocytic pathway of entry [69, 105]. This pathomechanism would also explain the results of a phase II, placebo-controlled, randomized, double-blind trial for the evaluation of a vaccine consisting of recombinant CMV envelope

Table 6.2 Human cytomegalovirus vaccines according to Schleiss et al. [102]

CMV vaccines currently undergoing evaluation in clinical trials	
Category	Status
V160-001 replication-defective vaccine	Phase I studies fully enrolled and data currently under analysis
PADRE-pp65-CMV fusion peptide vaccines ± CpG DNA adjuvant	Phase I studies currently ongoing
Modified vaccinia virus Ankara (MVA) "triplex" vaccine	Phase I study finished
gB/pp65 lymphocytic choriomeningitis virus (LCMV)-vector bivalent vaccine	Status not specified
gB/pp65/IE1 trivalent DNA vaccine; gB/pp65 bivalent DNA vaccine	Both (bivalent and trivalent) vaccine evaluated in phase I studies; phase III study of bivalent vaccine ongoing
Enveloped virus-like particle (eVLP) vaccine	Phase I study finished

glycoprotein B with MF59 adjuvant. Vaccine efficacy was found to be 50% on the basis of infection rates per 100 person-years [106]. Compared to the results of passive immunization to prevent transplacental CMV transmission [75], to date active immunization would be less efficient than passive immunization. Of course one has to keep in mind that the study design is not comparable between these two trials.

Nevertheless, the most fascinating result of the vaccination study was lowering the rate of maternal infection and reducing the transplacental CMV transmission, i.e., vaccine is superior to placebo [107, 108].

At the same time that these subunit-based approaches move forward, continued optimization of the immunogenicity of live, attenuated CMV vaccines was reported [109, 110], and others require further studies [111]. An excellent overview on recent strategies for the development of an HCMV vaccine was given by Schleiss et al. [102].

Despite some significant challenges, there are good reasons for being optimistic about the prospect of developing vaccines against cytomegalovirus. Now, the major obstacles for a human CMV vaccine will be difficulties associated with the design and execution of efficacy trials [100, 112].

References

1. Grosse SD, Dollard S, Ross DS, Cannon M (2009) Newborn screening for congenital cytomegalovirus: options for hospital-based and public health programs. J Clin Virol 46S: S32–S36
2. Schlesinger Y (2007) Routine screening for CMV in pregnancy: opening the pandora box? Isr Med Assoc J 9:395–397
3. Cahill AG, Odibo AO, Stamilio DM, Macones GA (2009) Screening and treating for primary cytomegalovirus infection in pregnancy: where do we stand? A decision-analytic and economic analysis. Am J Obstet Gynecol 201:466.e1–466.e7
4. Demmler-Harrison GJ (2009) J Clin Virol 46S:S1–S5
5. Fowler KB, Pass RF (2006) Risk factors for congenital cytomegalovirus infection in the offspring of young women: exposure to young children and recent onset of sexual activity. Pediatrics 118:e286–e292
6. Adler SP, Finney JW, Manganello AM, Best AM (2004) Prevention of child-to-mother transmission of cytomegalovirus among pregnant women. J Pediatr 145:485–491
7. Marshall BC, Adler SP (2009) The frequency of pregnancy and exposure to cytomegalovirus (CMV) infections among women with a young child in day care. Am J Obstet Gynecol 200 (2):163.e1–163.e5
8. Jeon J, Victor M, Adler SP, Arwady A, Demmler G, Fowler K, Goldfarb J, Keyserling H, Massoudi M, Richards K, Staras SAS, Cannon MJ (2006) Knowledge and awareness of congenital cytomegalovirus among women. Infect Dis Obstet Gynecol 2006:1–7
9. Cannon MJ, Westbrook K, Levis D, Schleiss MR, Thackeray R, Pass RF (2012) Awareness of and behaviors related to child-to-mother transmission of cytomegalovirus. Prev Med 54(5): 351–357
10. Harvey J, Dennis CL (2008) Hygiene interventions for prevention of cytomegalovirus infection among childbearing women: systematic review. J Adv Nurs 63(5):440–450
11. Valoup-Fellous C, Picone O, Cordier AG, Parent-du-Chatelet I, Senat MV, Frydman R, Grangeot-Keros L (2009) Does hygiene counselling have an impact on the rate of CMV

primary infection during pregnancy? Results of a 3-year prospective study in French hospital. J Clin Virol 46S:S49–S53
12. Pass RF, Arav-Boger R (2018) Maternal and fetal cytomegalovirus infection: diagnosis, management, and prevention. F1000Res 7:255
13. Revello MG, Tibaldi C, Masuelli G et al (2015) Prevention of primary cytomegalovirus infection in pregnancy. EBioMedicine 2:1205–1210
14. van Zuylen WJ, Hamilton ST, Naing Z, Hall B, Shand A, Rawlinson WD (2014) Congenital cytomegalovirus infection: clinical presentation, epidemiology, diagnosis and prevention. Obstet Med 7(4):140–146
15. Stowell JD, Forlin-Passoni D, Radford K et al (2014) Cytomegalovirus survival and transferability and the effectiveness of common hand-washing agents against cytomegalovirus on live human hands. Appl Environ Microbiol 80(2):455–461
16. Burny W, Liesnard C, Donner C, Marchant A (2004) Epidemiology, pathogenesis and prevention of congenital cytomegalovirus infection. Expert Rev Anti-Infect Ther 2(6): 881–894
17. Mercorelli B, Sinigalia E, Loregian A, Palu G (2008) Human cytomegalovirus DNA replication: antiviral targets and drugs. Rev Med Virol 18:177–210
18. Fiddian P, Sabin CA, Griffiths PD (2002) Valacyclovir provides optimum acyclovir exposure for prevention of cytomegalovirus and related outcomes after organ transplantation. J Infect Dis 186(Suppl 1):S110–S115
19. Talarico CL, Burnette TC, Miller WH et al (1999) Acyclovir is phosphorylated by the human cytomegalovirus UL97 protein. Antimicrob Agents Chemother 43(8):1941–1946
20. Nigro G, Sali E, Anceschi MM, Mazzocco M, Maranghi L, Clerico A, Castello MA (2004) Foscarnet therapy for congenital cytomegalovirus liver fibrosis following prenatal ascites. J Matern Fetal Neonatal Med 15(5):325–329
21. Nassetta L, Kimberlin D, Whitley R (2009) Treatment of congenital cytomegalovirus infection: implications for future therapeutic strategies. J Antimicrob Chemother 63:862–867
22. Marshall BC, Koch WC (2009) Antivirals for cytomegalovirus infection in neonates and infants: focus on pharmacokinetics, formulations, dosing, and adverse events. Paediatr Drugs 11(5):309–321
23. Trang JM, Kidd L, Gruber W, Storch G, Demmler G, Jacobs R, Dankner W, Starr S, Pass R, Stagno S, Alford C, Song SJ, Whitley RJ, Sommadossi JP (1993) Linear single-dose pharmacokinetics of ganciclovir in newborns with congenital cytomegalovirus infection. Clin Pharmacol Ther 53:15–21
24. Kimberlin DW, Acosta EP, Sanchez PJ, Sood S, Agrawal V, Homans J, Jacobs RF, Lang D, Romero JR, Grifin J, Cloud GA, Lakeman FD, Whitley RJ (2008) Pharmacokinetic and pharmacodynamic assessment of oral valganciclovir in the treatment of symptomatic congenital cytomegalovirus disease. J Infect Dis 197:836–845
25. Galli L, Novelli A, Chiappini E, Gervaso P, Cassetta MI, Fallani S, Martino M (2007) Valganciclovir for congenital CMV infection: a pilot study on plasma concentration in newborns and infants. J Pediatr Infect Dis 26(5):451–453
26. Jacquemard F, Yamamoto M, Costa JM, Romand S, Jaqz-Aigrain E, Dejean A, Daffos F, Ville Y (2007) Maternal administration of valaciclovir in symptomatic intrauterine cytomegalovirus infection. BJOG 114:1113–1121
27. Pacifici GM (2005) Transfer of antivirals across the human placenta. Early Hum Dev 81: 647–654
28. Leruez-Ville M, Ghout I, Bussières L et al (2016) In utero treatment of congenital cytomegalovirus infection with valacyclovir in a multicentre, open-label, phase II study. Am J Obstet Gynecol 215:462.e1–462.e10
29. Seidel V, Feiterna-Sperling C, Siedentopf JP et al (2017) Intrauterine therapy of cytomegalovirus infection with valganciclovir: review of the literature. Med Microbiol Immunol 206: 347–354
30. Rawlinson WD, Boppana SB, Fowler KB et al (2017) Congenital cytomegalovirus infection in pregnancy and the neonate: consensus recommendations for prevention, diagnosis, and therapy. Lancet Infect Dis 17:e177–e188

31. Rezanka E, Ploier R, Emhofer B, Emhofer J (1993) Congenital, generalized cytomegalovirus infection. Follow-up and therapeutic strategy with ganciclovir. Padiatr Padol 28(6):153–155
32. Junker AK, Matheson D, Tingle AT, Thomas EE (1991) Immune responses after ganciclovir and immunoglobulin therapy of infants. J Pediatr Infect Dis 10(3):256–258
33. Muntean W, Lackner H, Stünzner D, Ebner F (1989) 9 Wochen alter Säugling mit konnataler Zytomegalievirusinfection und Therapie mit Ganciclovir. Wien Klin Wochenschr 101: 554–557
34. Nigro G, Scholz H, Bartmann U (1994) Ganciclovir therapy for symptomatic congenital cytomegalovirus infection in infants: a two-regimen experience. J Pediatr 124:318–322
35. Whitley RJ, Cloud G, Gruber W, Storch GA, Demmler GJ, Jacobs RF, Dankner W, Spector SA, Starr S, Pass RF, Stagno S, Britt WJ, Alford C, Soong SJ, Zhou XJ, Sherrill L, FitzGerald JM, Sommadossi JP (1997) Ganciclovir treatment of symptomatic congenital cytomegalovirus infection: results of a phase II study. J Infect Dis 175:1080–1086
36. Halwachs-Baumann G, Genser B, Pailer S, Engele H, Rosegger H, Schalk A, Kessler HH, Truschnig-Wilders M (2002) Human cytomegalovirus load in various body fluids of congenitally infected newborns. J Clin Virol 25(Suppl 3):S81–S87
37. Michaels MG, Greenberg DP, Sabo DL, Wald ER (2003) Treatment of children with congenital cytomegalovirus infection with ganciclovir. Pediatr Infect Dis J 22:504–505
38. Kimberlin DW, Lin CY, Sanches PJ, Demmler GJ, Dankner W, Shelton M, Jacobs RF, Vaudry W, Pass RF, Kiell JM, Soong SJ, Whitley RJ (2003) Effect of ganciclovir therapy on hearing in symptomatic congenital cytomegalovirus disease involving the central nervous system: a randomized, controlled trial. J Pediatr 143:16–25
39. Kimberlin DW, Jester PM, Sánchez PJ et al (2015) Valganciclovir for symptomatic congenital cytomegalovirus disease. N Engl J Med 372(10):933–943
40. Oliver SE, Cloud G a, Sanchez PJ, Demmler GJ, Dankner W, Shelton M, Jacobs RF, Vaudry W, Pass RF, Soong SJ, Whitley RJ, Kimberlin DW (2009) Neurodevelopmental outcomes following ganciclovir therapy in symptomatic congenital cytomegalovirus infections involving the central nervous system. J Clin Virol 46S:S22–S26
41. Weng YH, Chu SM, Lien RI, Chou YH, Lin TY (2003) Clinical experience with ganciclovir and anti-cytomegalovirus immunoglobulin treatment for a severe case of congenital cytomegalovirus infection. Chang Gung Med J 26:128–132
42. Shoji K, Ito N, Ito Y, Inoue N, Adachi S, Fujimaru T, Nakamura T, Nishina S, Azuma N, Saitoh A (2010) Is a 6-week course of ganciclovir therapy effective for chorioretinitis in infants with congenital cytomegalovirus infection? J Pediatr 157(2):331–333
43. Yilmaz CD, Vardar F (2011) Effect on hearing of oral valganciclovir for asymptomatic congenital cytomegalovirus infection. J Trop Pediatr 57(2):132–134
44. Amir J, Wolf DG, Levy I (2010) Treatment of symptomatic congenital cytomegalovirus infection with intravenous ganciclovir followed by long-term oral valganciclovir. Eur J Pediatr 169(9):1061–1067. https://doi.org/10.1007/s00431-010-1176-9
45. Gandhi RS, Fernandez-Alvarez JR, Rabe H (2010) Management of congenital cytomegalovirus infection: an evidence-based approach. Acta Paediatr 99:509–515
46. Luck S, Sharland M, Griffiths P (2007) Ganciclovir therapy for neonates with congenital cytomegalovirus infection. Eur J Pediatr 166:633–634
47. Smets K, De Coen K, Dhooge I, Standaert L, Laroche S, Mahieu L, Logghe N, Cossey V, Boudewyns A (2006) Selecting neonates with congenital cytomegalovirus infection for ganciclovir therapy. Eur J Pediatr 165:885–890
48. Prober C g, Enright AM (2003) Congenital cytomegalovirus (CMV) infections: hats off to Alabama. J Pediatr 143:4–6
49. Michaels MG (2007) Treatment of congenital cytomegalovirus: where are we now? Expert Rev Anti-Infect Ther 5(3):441–448
50. Demmler GJ (2003) Congenital cytomegalovirus infection treatment. Pediatr Infect Dis J 22: 1003–1006
51. Dahle AJ, fowler KB, Wright JD, Boppana SB, Britt WJ, Pass RF (2000) Longitudinal investigation of hearing disorders in children with congenital cytomegalovirus. J Am Acad Audiol 11(5):283–290

52. Fowler KB, McCollister FP, Dahle AJ, Boppana S, Britt WJ, Pass RF (1997) Progressive and fluctuating sensorineural hearing loss in children with asymptomatic congenital cytomegalovirus infection. J Pediatr 130:624–630
53. Lackner A, Acham A, Alborno T, Moser M, Engele H, Raggam RB, Halwachs-Baumann G, Kapitan M, Walch C (2009) Effect on hearing of ganciclovir therapy for asymptomatic congenital cytomegalovirus infection: four to 10 year follow up. J Laryngol Otol 123(4): 391–396
54. James SH, Kimberlin DW (2016) Advances in the prevention and treatment of congenital cytomegalovirus infection. Curr Opin Pediatr 28(1):81–85
55. James SH, Kimberlin DW, Whitley RJ (2009) Antiviral therapy for herpesvirus central nervous system infections: neonatal herpes simplex virus infection, herpes simplex encephalitis, and congenital cytomegalovirus infection. Antivir Res 83:207–213
56. Clark AL, Gall SA (1997) Clinical uses of intravenous immunoglobulin in pregnancy. Am J Obstet Gynecol 176:241–253
57. Clark AL (1999) Clinical uses of intravenous immunoglobulin in pregnancy. Clin Obstet Gynecol 42(2):368–380
58. Adler SP, Nigro G (2009) Findings and conclusions from CMV hyperimmune globulin treatment trials. J Clin Virol 46S:S54–S57
59. Keller MA, Stiehm ER (2000) Passive immunity I prevention and treatment of infectious diseases. Clin Microbial Rev 13(4):602–614
60. Chang MH (2007) Hepatitis B virus infection. Semin Fetal Neonatal Med 12:160–167
61. Rhiner J, Pfister R, Tschopp YN, Bucher H (2007) Ul. Selective immunisation strategy to protect newborns at risk for transmission of hepatitis B: retrospective audit of vaccine uptake. Swiss Med Wkly 137:531–535
62. (1990) Protection against viral hepatitis. Recommendations of the Immunization Practices Advisory Committee (ACIP). MMWR Recomm Rep 9:1–26
63. Heininger U, Vaudaux B, Nidecker M, Pfister RE, Posfay-Barbe KM, Bachofner M, Hoigne I, Gnehm HE (2010) Evaluation of the compliance with recommended procedures in newborns exposed to HBsAg-positive mothers: a multicenter collaborative study. Pediatr Infect Dis J 29(3):248–250
64. (1990) NIH Consensus Conference. Intravenus immunoglobulin. Prevention and treatment of disease. J Am Med Assoc 264:3189–3193
65. Lories RJU, Maertens JA, Ceuppens JL, Peetermans WE (2000) The use of polyclonal intravenous immunoglobulins in the prevention and treatment of infectious diseases. Acta Clin Belg 55(3):163–169
66. Von Muralt G, Sidiropoulos D (1988) Prenatal and postnatal prophylaxis of infections in preterm neonates. Pediatr Infect Dis J 7(5):S072–S078
67. Jauniaux E, Jurkovic D, Gulbis B, Liesnard C, Lees C, Campbell S (1995) Materno-fetal immunoglobulin transfer and passive immunity during the first trimester of human pregnancy. Hum Reprod 10(2):3297–3300
68. Adler SP, Starr SE, Plotkin SA, Hempfling SH, Buis J, Manning ML, Best AM (1995) Immunity induced by primary human cytomegalovirus infection protects against secondary infection among women of childbearing age. J Infect Dis 171(1):26–32
69. Cui X, Meza BP, Adler SP, McVoy MA (2008) Cytomegalovirus vaccines fail to induce epithelial entry neutralizing antibodies comparable to natural infection. Vaccine 26(45): 5760–5766
70. Cekinovic D, Golemac M, Pugel EP, Tomac J, Cicin-Sain L, Slavuljica I, Bradford R, Misch S, Winkler TH, Mach M, Britt WJ, Jonjic S (2008) Passive immunization reduces murine cytomegalovirus-induced brain pathology in newborn mice. J Virol 82(24): 12172–12180
71. Negishi H, Yamada H, Hirayama E, Okuyama K, Sagawa T, Matsumoto Y, Fujimoto S (1998) Intraperitoneal administration of cytomegalovirus hyperimmunoglobulin to the cytomegalovirus infected fetus. J Perinatol 18(6):466–469

72. Breindl A, Lassmann R (1989) Zytomegalie-Infektion bei Zwillingsschwangerschaft – Reversibilität eines Hydrops fetalis nach Behandlung mit Humanimmunglobulin (Cytotect®). Gynecologie 12:339–341
73. Moxley K, Knudtson EJ (2008) Resolution of hydrops secondary to cytomegalovirus after naternal and fetal treatment with human cytomegalovirus hyperimmune globulin. Obstet Gynecol 111(2):524–526
74. Nigro G, La Torre R, Anceschi MM, Mazzocco M, Cosmi EV (1999) Hyperimmunoglobulin therapy for a twin fetus with cytomegalovirus infection and growth restriction. Am J Obstet Gynecol 180:1222–1226
75. Nigro G, Adler SP, La Torre R, Best AM (2005) Passive immunization during pregnancy for congenital cytomegalovirus infection. N Engl J Med 29:1350–1362
76. La Torre R, Nigro G, Mazzocco M, Best AB, Adler SP (2006) Placental enlargement in women with primary maternal cytomegalovirus infection is associated with fetal and neonatal disease. Clin Infect Dis 43:994–1000
77. Schleiss MR (2006) The role of the placenta in the pathogenesis of congenital cytomegalovirus infection: is the benefit of cytomegalovirus immune globulin for the newborn mediated through improved placental health and function? Clin Infect Dis 43:1001–1003
78. Duff P (2005) Immunotherapy for congenital cytomegalovirus infection. N Engl J Med 353: 1402–1404
79. Silverman NS, Puliyanda D, Lehman D (2005) Passive immunization against cytomegalovirus during pregnancy. N Engl J Med 353:2818
80. Carbillon L (2005) Passive immunization against cytomegalovirus during pregnancy. N Engl J Med 353:2828–2818
81. Revello MG (2005) Passive immunization against cytomegalovirus during pregnancy. N Engl J Med 353:2819
82. Nigro G, Adler S (2005) Passive immunization against cytomegalovirus during pregnancy. N Engl J Med 353:2819–2820
83. Adler SP (2008) The importance of cytomegalovirus-specific antibodies for the prevention of fetal cytomegalovirus infection or disease. Herpesviridae 15(2):24–27
84. Adler SP, Nigro G, Pereira L (2007) Recent advances in the prevention and treatment of congenital cytomegalovirus infections. Semin Perinatol 31:10–18
85. Nigro G (2009) Maternal-fetal cytomegalovirus infection: from diagnosis to therapy. J Matern Fetal Neonatal Med 22(2):169–174
86. Revello MG, Lazzarotto T, Guerra B et al (2014) A randomized trial of hyperimmune globulin to prevent congenital cytomegalovirus. N Engl J Med 370:1316–1326
87. Blázquez-Gamero D, Galindo Izquierdo A, Del Rosal T et al (2017) Prevention and treatment of fetal cytomegalovirus infection with cytomegalovirus hyperimmune globulin: a multicentre study in Madrid. J Matern Fetal Neonatal Med 26:1–9
88. Nigro G, Capretti I, Manganello AM, Best AM, Adler SP (2015) Primary maternal cytomegalovirus infections during pregnancy: association of CMV hyperimmune globulin with gestational age at birth and birth weight. J Matern Fetal Neonatal Med 28(2):168–171
89. Delle Chiaie L, Neuberger P, Vochem M, Lihs A, Karck U, Enders M (2018) No evidence of obstetrical adverse events after hyperimmune globulin application for primary cytomegalovirus infection in pregnancy: experience from a single centre. Arch Gynecol Obstet 297(6): 1389–1395. https://doi.org/10.1007/s00404-018-4703-y
90. Jückstock J, Rothenburger M, Friese K, Traunbüller F (2015) Passive immunization against congenital cytomegalovirus infection: current state of knowledge. Pharmacology 95:209–217
91. Visentin S, Manara R, Milanese L et al (2012) Early primary cytomegalovirus infection in pregnancy: maternal hyperimmunoglobulin therapy improves outcomes among infants at 1 year of age. CID 55:497–503
92. Pass RF, Burke RL (2002) Development of cytomegalovirus vaccines: prospects for prevention of congenital CMV infection. Semin Pediatr Infect Dis 13(3):196–204
93. Griffiths PD, McLean A, Emery VC (2001) Encouraging prospects for immunisation against primary cytomegalovirus infection. Vaccine 19:1356–1362

94. Schleiss MR, Bourne N, Jensen NJ, Bravo F, Bernstein DI (2000) Immunogenicity evaluation of DNA vaccines that target guinea pig cytomegalovirus proteins glycoprotein B and UL83. Viral Immunol 13(2):155–167
95. Pass RF, Duliege AM, Boppana S, Sekulovich R, Percell S, Britt W, Burke RL (1999) A subunit cytomegalovirus vaccine based on recombinant envelope glycoprotein B and a new adjuvant. J Infect Dis 180:970–975
96. Adler SP (1996) Current prospects for immunization against cytomegaloviral disease. Infect Agents Dis 5:29–35
97. Harrison CJ, Britt WJ, Chapman NM, Mullican J, Tracy S (1995) Reduced congenital cytomegalovirus (CMV) infection after maternal immunization with a guinea pig CMV glycoprotein before gestational primary CMV infection in the guinea pig model. J Infect Dis 172:1212–1220
98. Bourne N, Schleiss MR, Bravo FJ, Bernstein DI (2001) Preconception immunization with a cytomegalovirus (CMV) glycoprotein vaccine improves pregnancy outcome in a guinea pig model of congenital CMV infection. J Infect Dis 183:59–64
99. Schleiss MR (2009) Cytomegalovirus vaccines: at last, a major step forward. Herpesviridae 15:44–45
100. Adler SP (2008) Human CMV vaccine trials: what if CMV caused a rash? J Clin Virol 41: 231–236
101. Schleiss MR, Heineman TC (2005) Progress toward an elusive goal: current status of cytomegalovirus vaccines. Expert Rev Vaccines 4(3):381–406
102. Schleiss MR, Permar SR, Plotkin SA (2017) Progress toward development of a vaccine against congenital cytomegalovirus infection. Clin Vaccine Immunol 24(12):e00268–e00217
103. Schleiss M (2005) Progress in cytomegalovirus vaccine development. Herpesviridae 12(3): 66–75
104. Schleiss MR (2010) Cytomegalovirus vaccines and methods of production (WO20009049138): the emerging recognition of the importance of virus neutralization at the epithelial/endothelial interface. Expert Opin Ther Pat 20(4):597–602
105. Gerna G, Sarasini A, Patrone M, Percivalle E, Fiorina L, Campanini G, Gallina A, Baldanti F, Revello MG (2008) Human cytomegalovirus serum neutralizing antibodies block virus infection of endothelial/epithelial cells, but not fibroblasts, early during primary infection. J Gen Virol 89:853–865
106. Pass RF, Zhang C, Evans A, Simpson T, Andrews W, Huang ML, Corey L, Hill J, Davis E, Flanigan C, Cloud G (2009) Vaccine prevention of maternal cytomegalovirus infection. N Engl J Med 360(12):1191–1199
107. Dekker CL, Arvin AM (2009) One step closer to a CMV vaccine. N Engl J Med 360(12): 1250–1252
108. Pass RF (2009) Development and evidence for efficacy of CM glycoprotein B vaccine with MF59 adjuvant. J Clin Virol 46(Suppl 4):S73–S76. https://doi.org/10.1016/j.jcv.2009.07.002
109. Jacobson MA, Adler SP, Sinclair E, Black D, Smith A, Chu A, Moss RB, Wloch MK (2009) A CMV DNA vaccine primes for memory immune responses to live-attenuated CMV (Towne strain). Vaccine 15:1540–1548
110. Clumpler MM, Choi KY, McVoy MA, Schleiss MR (2009) A live guinea pig cytomegalovirus vaccine deleted of three putative immune evasion genes is highly attenuated but remains immunogenic in a vaccine/challenge model of congenital cytomegalovirus infection. Vaccine 27:4209–4218
111. Heineman TC, Schleiss M, Bernstein DI, Spaete RR, Yan L, Dukle G, Prichard M, Wang Z, Yan Q, Sharp MA, Klein N, Arvin AM, Kemble G (2006) A phase I study of 4 live, recombinant human cytomegalovirus Towne/Toledo chimeric vaccines. J Infect Dis 193: 1350–1360
112. Griffiths PD (2009) CMV vaccine trial endpoints. J Clin Virol 46S:S64–S67

7 How to Save Money: Congenital CMV Infection and the Economy

E. Walter, C. Brennig, V. Schöllbauer, and Gabriele Halwachs-Baumann

7.1 Introduction

Human cytomegalovirus (CMV) is the main cause of congenital virus infection in developed countries leading to psychomotor impairment, deafness and blindness. In Germany each year, estimated 6500 children are born with congenital cytomegalovirus (CMV) infection, causing estimated 40 deaths and leaving approximately 1200 children (primary infected and from seropositive women) with permanent disabilities such as hearing or vision loss or mental retardation. More children are affected by serious CMV-related disabilities than by several better-known childhood maladies, including Down syndrome [1].

The infection causes high disease burden and costs. The disease burden of congenital CMV infection is similar to that of congenital rubella before the introduction of rubella vaccination [2]. Since congenital CMV affects the very young, it results in lifetime morbidity. The direct and indirect annual economic costs of caring for these children are enormous. In the 1990s the estimated costs associated with CMV disease for the US health-care system amounted annually to 1.86 billion US dollars with more than 300,000 US dollars per child [2]. Porath and colleagues (1990) calculate for populations with lower seroprevalence (55–70%); for every 100,000 women immunised, more than 24 cases of symptomatic congenital CMV infection at birth and a similar number of cases with late sequelae (mainly deafness) would be prevented yearly. Such immunisation would result in a net annual saving of 2.5 million US dollars [3].

E. Walter (✉) · C. Brennig · V. Schöllbauer
IPF Institute for Pharmaeconomic Research, Vienna, Austria
e-mail: e.walter@ipf-ac.at; c.brennig@ipf-ac.at; v.schoellbauer@ipf-ac.at

G. Halwachs-Baumann
Department of Laboratory Medicine, Regional Hospital Steyr, Steyr, Austria
e-mail: gabriele.baumann@gespag.at

G. Halwachs-Baumann (ed.), *Congenital Cytomegalovirus Infection*,
https://doi.org/10.1007/978-3-319-98770-5_7

At present economic analyses in the field of diagnostic strategies are scarce. The reasons are manifold. In order to measure outcomes, it must be clear that the results of a diagnostic test and the actual health outcome are indirectly related. Diagnostic test results are intermediate outcomes; they influence but are not directly responsible for the health outcome of patients. Therefore diagnostic technologies differ from therapeutic medical technologies [4]. Diagnostic technologies certainly affect long-term outcomes in patients by forwarding information and, hence, can improve medical treatment. From the cost side, it must be considered that costs of a diagnostic strategy arise for the whole population tested. However, the benefits accrue only to a part of the total population. More importantly, cost/benefit relations have to be perceived from the perspective of policymakers where costs arise in the short term yet benefits occur in the future. In this respect, economic analysis of diagnostic tests differs from conventional health cost/benefit analysis and presents challenges to the health economist.

Congenital CMV is a prime target for prevention not only because of its substantial disease burden but also because biology and epidemiology of CMV suggest that there are ways to reduce viral transmission. Screening programs for pregnant women and newborns are widely discussed but have not been implemented by any public health authority in Europe so far [2]. However, a fair discussion on screening programs cannot be started without knowledge of the epidemiological and economic background.

The objective of this study was to estimate the total economic impact (lifetime direct and indirect costs based on deliveries p.a.) on society due to CMV infection based on incidences. Calculations were done for Germany, and adaptations for further countries are ongoing. Furthermore this study shows the positive monetary impact of screening (serologic testing and treatment in case of primary infection).

7.2 Methodology

To estimate the whole economic burden due to CMV infection, a cost-of-illness (COI) study (or synonym burden of illness) was adopted. Cost-of-illness studies measure the economic burden of a disease and estimate the maximum amount that could potentially be saved or gained if a disease was to be eradicated. This kind of study does not focus on a particular intervention and does not address any question regarding treatment efficacy or effectiveness.

At present, there are several methods for cost-of-illness studies. Akobundu et al. (2006) established a review and classified different existing methods for cost-of-illness studies [5], with four categories of cost-of-illness studies (see Table 7.1). In accordance, the present analysis uses the first method "Sum All Medical", i.e. all costs associated with CMV infection are collected and summed up.

Table 7.1 Categorisation of COI methods

COI method	Description
1. Sum_All Medical	Identify all patients with a diagnosis and sum costs
2. Sum_Diagnosis Specific	Identify all patients with a primary diagnosis and sum costs for treatments for that diagnosis
3. Matched Control	Identify all patients with a diagnosis and sum cost. Subtract out the average cost of the sample to find incremental costs for treatment; alternatively, subtract out the average cost of a matched cohort instead
4. Regression	Identify all patients with a diagnosis, complete a regression analysis, and indicate the individual ß for each diagnosis Identify all patients with a diagnosis, find a matched cohort (similar to a clinical trial), and complete a regression analysis to quantify the individual ß for each diagnosis – gold standard

Source: Akobundu et al. (2006)

7.2.1 Incidence-Based Approach

The approach used is incidence-based; that means it estimates lifetime costs and measures the costs of an illness from onset over lifetime. In general, there are two types of cost-of-illness studies: prevalence- and incidence-based. In the prevalence-based studies, only costs of resources used or losses incurred during the study, which usually were foregone within the time horizon of 1 year, are considered. Prevalence estimates are best suited for cost control and annual budget planning. Incidence-based COI studies evaluate lifetime costs and apply these costs to the year in which the disease arises. They require data on lifetime medical, morbidity and disability, foregone earnings and mortality costs, life expectancy, epidemiology and the natural history of sequelae for the incident cohort. The incidence-based approach is a suitable concept to analyse the socio-economic relevance of the maternal CMV infection during pregnancy. They are more useful, however, when evaluating a program since incidence-based data provide a baseline for new treatment intervention. Incidence-based data can also help decisions about prevention programs.

The incidence of CMV infection in general varies according to socio-economic background. In the United States, the seropositivity rate is 50–60% for women of middleclass background, but it is 70–80% for those from lower socio-economic sectors. In Europe, 45% (range 43–73%) of pregnant women are seropositive at the beginning of pregnancy. The risk of seroconversion during pregnancy, which on average is 2.0–2.5%, ranges from 0.47% to 12.9%. The rate of congenital infection resulting from primary maternal infection is about 30%, ranging from 15% to 50%, and after a recurrent infection (reactivation or reinfection), it is 0.15–1%. Ten percent of congenitally infected infants have congenital CMV syndrome, whereas 90% are asymptomatic at birth; however, 10–15% of the latter are at risk of developing a multitude of developmental abnormalities such as sensorineural hearing loss, chorioretinitis or neurologic deficits. Among the most severely affected infants, mortality may be as high as 30%. More than 90% of the infants surviving CMV disease have complications later on, such as hearing loss, mental retardation, delay in psychomotor development, chorioretinitis, optic atrophy, seizures, expressive language delays and learning disabilities [6].

Epidemiological data differ among countries. According to Halwachs-Baumann, the prevalence of CMV in Europe is 0.04–0.49%, resp., and 0.22–2.2% in North America [7]. The model is based on epidemiological data published by Halwachs-Baumann et al. o.J [8].

Figure 7.1 shows the epidemiological structure of the CMV burden of disease model. It exhibits the total number of births per year (n = 700,000) in Germany and distinguishes between pregnant women without prior CMV contact and seropositive

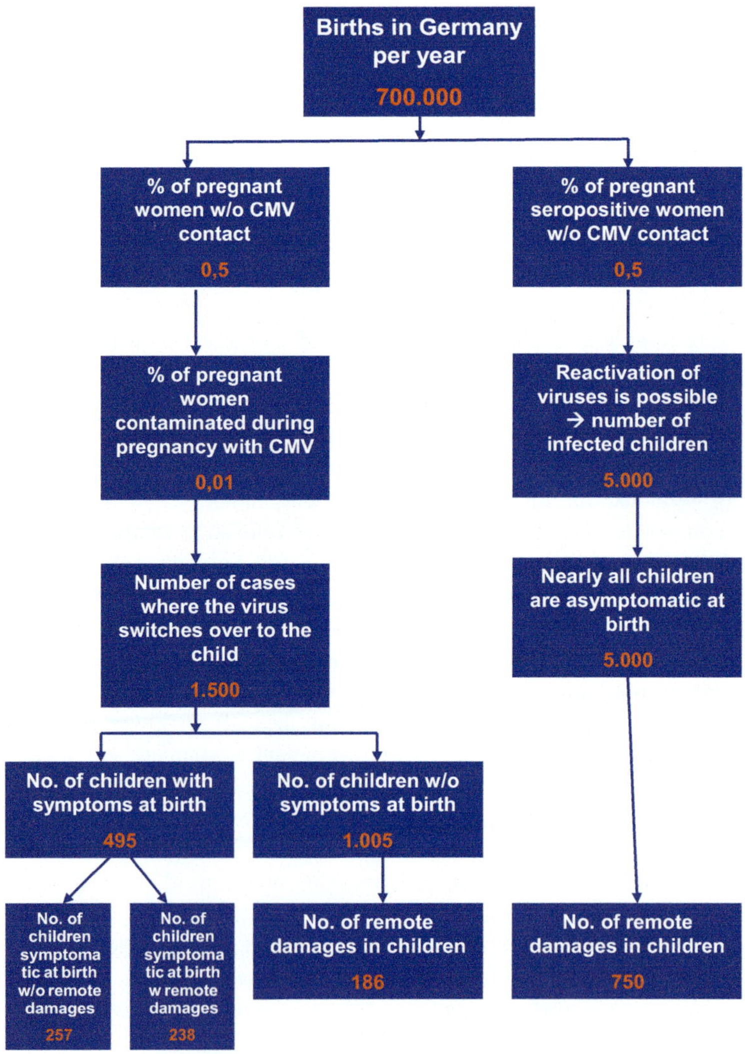

Fig. 7.1 Epidemiological structure based on Incidence. Source: Halwachs-Baumann et al. o.J

women without CMV contact. The path of pregnant women without prior CMV contact differentiates between the number of newborns with symptoms at birth (those are furthermore divided in symptomatic children without remote damages and in those with additional remote damages) and the number of newborns without symptoms at birth but with remote damages. The path of pregnant seropositive women includes the number of children with remote damages. For incidences of sequelae of symptomatic and asymptomatic children at birth as well as of sequelae of children with remote damages, see Tables 7.2 and 7.3.

Tables 7.2 and 7.3 show the incidences of sequelae for symptomatic children at birth as well as for children asymptomatic at birth. The burden of disease model allows the appearance of more than one symptom. The incidences for asymptomatic

Table 7.2 Symptoms after birth resp. within the first postnatal month

Symptoms after birth respective within the first postnatal month	Incidence/base case (%)	Source
Petechiae	0.44	[7]
IUGH (intrauterine growth retardation)	0.36	[7]
Icterus	0.34	[7]
Hepatosplenomegalies	0.33	[7]
Hearing loss	0.40	[9, 10]
Intracranial calcification	0.28	[7]
Microcephalus	0.28	[7]
Inexplicable abnormalities	0.23	[7]
Pneumonia	0.08	[7]
Haemolytic anaemia	0.08	[7]
Chorioretinitis	0.07	[7]
Convulsions	0.07	[7]
Prematurity	0.05	[7]
Birth weight (>2500 g)	0.03	[7]
Hepatitis	0.02	[7]
Hydrocephalus	0.002	[7]
Death	0.06	[7]

Table 7.3 Symptoms: sequelae (later than the first postnatal month)

Symptoms: sequelae (later than the first postnatal month)	Incidence/base case (%)	Source
Hearing loss	0.22	[7]
Mental retardation	0.22	[7]
Cerebral paresis	0.04	[11]
Convulsions	0.02	[11]
Developmental disorder	0.06	[11]
Chorioretinitis	0.02	[7]
Microcephalus	0.014	[7]
Death	0.004	[7]

children at birth are used for the calculation of cost of remote damages due to CMV infection.

7.2.2 Cost Calculation

To calculate the total costs associated with CMV Infection, health economics generally distinguish three categories: direct, indirect and intangible costs. Direct costs cover all costs which are directly associated with the illness, including inpatient and outpatient costs, procedures, diagnostic tests and medication. Indirect costs quantify the estimated loss of income as a result of illness, disability or death. Intangible costs include nonquantifiable costs associated with physical and emotional pain and suffering. In order to estimate the disease burden due to CMV infection in Germany, both direct and indirect costs have to be analysed. Recourse use (i.e. the type and frequency of medical goods and services rendered to the patient) and monetary value (prices, tariffs and/or opportunity costs) for each unit of medical goods and services were used to calculate the direct costs. Data on resource use was determined by literature and expert opinion. All resource data were externally validated by experts. Indirect costs were calculated using human productivity as substitute to estimate the effect of CMV infection for parents and affected children on society in monetary terms. The human capital approach is commonly used since human health and life cannot easily be expressed in monetary values [12]. Indirect costs include the reduced productivity of parents due to care for their affected children and the lost productivity of the affected due to their incapability to work. To calculate the indirect costs, data from the literature were used. All costs represent data from 2008.

The burden of disease study was conducted from a societal perspective, because all costs in relation to CMV infection and sequelae are considered.

The cost-of-illness study uses lifetime horizons. A lifetime horizon requires discounting. According to German Guidelines for Health Economic Analyses, a discount rate of 5% was applied [13].

This cost-of-illness study uses the life expectancy published by the "Deutsches Bundesamt", 79.57 years [14]. It is assumed and acknowledged by experts that the majority of the children, except those suffering from blindness, deafness or mental retardation, do reach this average life expectancy. For the abovementioned sequelae, reduced life expectancy data derived from the WHO was used [15]. Table 7.4 shows statistical life expectancy data.

To estimate the socio-economic consequences of CMV infection from a societal perspective, a Microsoft Excel model was built. This model includes direct and indirect costs of all affected infants concerned over the lifetime. Costs were collected bottom-up and have been discounted.

The economic analysis was conducted in accordance with the "German Recommendations on Health Economic Evaluation: Third and Updated Version of the Hanover Consensus" [13].

Table 7.4 Life expectancy

	Life expectancy
Life expectancy at birth	79.57
Life expectancy at birth (2 years reduced, remote sequelae)	77.57
Life expectancy at birth (8 years reduced, remote sequelae, mental retardation)	71.57
Life expectancy at birth (blindness HR 0.5, remote sequelae)	37.79
Life expectancy at birth (blindness HR 0.5)	39.79
Life expectancy at birth (hearing loss HR 0.83, 2 years reduced, remote sequelae)	64.04
Life expectancy at birth (hearing loss HR 0.83)	66.04

Source: Deutsches Bundesamt, WHO, IPF own calculations

Table 7.5 Direct and indirect cost data

Direct cost	Indirect cost
⇨ Direct medical cost » Consultations (EBM catalogue 2008) » Inpatient cost (G-DRG-catalogue) » Medication (health insurance prices) » Treatment cost (EBM catalogue 2008)	⇨ Impact of care on job situation of parents (until the children's age of 18) ⇨ Absenteeism ⇨ Nursing leave ⇨ Human capital of dead people ⇨ Cost of blindness (from the age of 18 on) ⇨ Cost of schools for blind, deaf and handicapped people (Halwachs-Baumann, Preuss et al., BMI Deutschland) ⇨ Cost of nursing homes for severe handicapped people (AOK 2009)

Source: IPF own depiction

7.2.3 Cost of Sequelae

The total costs per patient are a function of both the quantity of a given resource used and its unit cost. The costs of sequelae due to CMV infection are derived from various sources.

Table 7.5 exhibits the components of direct and indirect cost used in the model. Direct medical costs are derived from a number of publicly available sources like the EBM tariff catalogue as well as the G-DRG catalogue and official price lists for the German health insurances. Indirect cost represents statistical and published data as well as own calculations. When it was necessary, prices were adjusted to 2008 prices using the consumer price index.

7.2.3.1 Direct Cost Data

Direct Cost data represent direct medical cost like consultation cost, inpatient cost, medication cost and diagnostic and treatment cost. Costs per symptom were derived on a yearly basis, except of nonrecurring symptoms after birth like prematurity, pneumonia, icterus, etc., which were captured per event in the first year of event.

Data on the resource use of CMV infection was collected in two steps. First, the medical resources were derived by country-specific literature (e.g. disease-specific guidelines). In a second step, this literature review was verified by experts (Dr. Heidemarie Engele, University Clinic Graz, Austria; Prim. Dr. Johannes Fellinger and Dr. Daniel Holzinger, Hospital Barmherzige Brüder Linz, Austria) concerning clinical practice as external validation. This was necessary because the utilisation of medical resources often differs between health-care systems, medical tradition, ease of access and availability.

Every symptomatic CMV-infected child will stay in hospital for about 14 days. Inpatient costs are generally assessed using the German DRG catalogue. The point value represents a weighted average of all federal states of Germany [16]. Cost for doctor visits, lab tests and treatment costs are costs from the German EBM catalogue. The cost of medication represents the health insurance price. Over-the-counter medication are valued with the public price. The cost of medical devices, e.g. hearing device and walking stick, is derived from tariffs of the national health insurance (AOK 2008 [17]). The cost for physiotherapy, logo therapy, etc. is evaluated using the EBM catalogue. Direct cost of death is estimated by using the cost for a 14-day-inpatient stay at the intensive care unit for newborns.

In general the resource use is derived from literature validated by expert opinion. The following cost positions include cost for special devices:

- Cost of blindness: Guide dog (assumed life expectancy: 10 years; 1.5% of blind people own a guide dog) [18] and walking stick (once per year paid by health insurance).
- Cost of deafness/hearing impairment: Cochlear Implant (once per lifetime), hearing device incl. battery (once per 6 years), battery for cochlear implant (once per week) and logopaedic therapy (every 2 weeks until the age of 18 years).
- Cost of inexplicable abnormalities: due to missing data, the cost and resource use of these sequelae were derived using average cost and resource use of mental retardation and developmental disorder.
- Cost of mental retardation: in addition to out- and inpatient treatments, patients need according to their stage of illness different treatments, like physio- (avg. 1/month, from the age of 8 years on: 1/year), ergo- (avg. 1/month, from the age of 8 years on: 1/year) and logo therapy (avg. 1/month, from the age of 8 years on: 1/year) in the group of 0–50% mentally handicapped children; like physio- (avg. 1/month, from the age of 2–4 years on: 1/quarter, from the age of 5 years on 2/years), ergo- (avg. 1/month, from the age of 2–4 years on: 1/quarter, from the age of 5 years on 2/years) and logo therapy (avg. 1/month, from the age of 2–4 years on: 1/quarter, from the age of 5 years on 2/years), in the group of >50% mentally handicapped children.
- Cost of developmental disorder: in addition to out- and inpatient treatments, patients need according to their stage of illness different treatments, like physio- (avg. 1/quarter), ergo- (avg. 1/quarter) and logo therapy (avg. 1/quarter).

Tables 7.6 and 7.7 show the resource use and cost per sequelae and year/event for the first year of symptomatic children and the total cost per sequelae for lifetime.

Table 7.6 Direct costs of sequelae of symptomatic children

Sequelae	Total direct cost per lifetime
Inpatient therapy of CMV after birth	4,286.40 (cost for the first year)
Visual impairment/chorioretinitis[a]	1,258.47
Blindness until the age of 18 [18]	33,088.59
Hearing loss [17]	91,549.48
Purpura/petechiae[a]	Included in inpatient therapy of CMV after birth
Hepatosplenomegaly[a]	Included in inpatient therapy of CMV after birth
Microcephalus[a]	9.23
Convulsions [19]	132,845.17
Pneumonia[a]	2887.17
Haemolytic anaemia[a]	1900.79
Icterus[a]	4404.20
Hydrocephalus[a]	76,400.63
Intracranial calcification[a]	1349.94
Prematurity	1035.38
Birth weight <2500 g	916.47
Hepatitis	239.49
IUGH	885.07
Inexplicable abnormalities	53,535.17[b]
Cost of death [7]	10,670.31

[a]Expert opinion
[b]Avg. value of neurological abnormalities of asymptomatic children at birth
Source: IPF own calculations

Table 7.7 Direct costs of sequelae of asymptomatic children

Sequelae	Total direct cost per lifetime
Mental retardation [20]	12,105.96
Visual impairment/Chorioretinitis[a]	1221.59
Blindness until the age of 18 [18]	33,085.89
Hearing loss [19]	89,180.34
Microcephalus[a]	6.92
Cerebral paresis	112,687.06
Convulsions [19]	128,889.03
Developmental disorder [20]	27,751.10
Cost of death	10,670.31

[a]Expert opinion
Source: IPF own calculations

7.2.3.2 Indirect Cost Data

The indirect cost data include the following positions:

- Impact of care on job situation of parents (until the children's age of 18 years)
- Absenteeism
- Nursing leave

- Human capital of dead people
- Cost of schools for blind, deaf and handicapped people
- Cost of nursing homes for severe handicapped people
- Cost of blindness (from the age of 18 on)

To investigate the change of job situation of parents with CMV-infected children with sequelae, a study from Lange et al. (2004) was used which analyses the burden and the financial and professional consequences for mothers and fathers after the onset of diabetes in their children. According to experts, children with CMV infection and sequelae have a comparable nursing effort (rather more depending on the kind of sequelae). Hence, we used a conservative assumption for the study [21].

The study from Lange et al. (2004) includes 580 German families with 583 children with diabetes type 1. The study expresses the German working situation of young parents. Before the onset of disease in their children, 93% of the fathers worked full-time; thereafter 4% changed their employment. Twenty-two percent of mothers worked at onset full time and 38% part time; thereafter 31% reduced their working time or stopped working. Negative financial consequences were present in 44% of the families [21] (see Table 7.8).

Production losses were valued with the human capital approach according to health economic guidelines [13], where the production of a person is valued at the market price (in this case, the sex-specific average gross salary). For short-term nursing leave, labour costs were adjusted to patients' working absenteeism. In Germany, 20 days at nursing leaves are permitted per year. We assume that in the case of CMV-infected children, parents have to use all permitted days. For the long-term changing job situation (stop working or part-time working instead of full time) due to caring children, the reduced sex-specific average gross salary for the national average annual working years by sex was used. Indirect costs for dead people represent their human capital up to the average retirement age. This method of estimation of indirect costs is the most commonly used one in economic studies; although it has been suggested that it may overestimate costs, as particularly in times of unemployment, a worker would be rapidly replaced, and hence no production loss

Table 7.8 Impact of care on job situation of parents

	Age of child		
Working situation at time of diagnosis	< 6 years	6–10 years	11–14 years
Housewife	50%	38.6%	24.2%
Part-time	32.9%	35.9%	50.3%
Full-time	17.1%	25.5%	25.5%
Consequences	< 6 years	6–10 years	11–14 years
Termination of employment	20.50%	12.00%	6.60%
Career changes	32.50%	25.50%	17.00%
Changes of career planning	44.10%	34.50%	21.10%

Source: Lange et al. (2004)

would occur. A different method of calculation (friction cost method) has therefore been proposed, but is not generally used.

Costs for special schools for handicapped children were also included in the indirect cost calculation. It is necessary to distinguish between a mild and severe handicap. Mild disabled children with normal intelligence are able to attend regular schools supported by a special mobile teacher. Costs for a mobile teacher are valued with the gross salary derived from the pay regulation from the Ministry of Internal Affairs. Indirect costs for special schools for blind and deaf pupils were valued with the annual costs per child and were derived by literature. School attendance is not only associated with compulsory education but also with disability-specific education.

It is assumed that one third of severe handicapped persons (after age of 18 years) need care in nursing homes. This assumption is based on expert opinions.

In economic terms, indirect costs of blindness from the age of 18 years on depend on cost incurred by the blind person due to loss of productivity, and indirect cost incurred by the family, nursing expenses and costs for nursing homes of the blind person. To estimate these costs of blindness for Germany, we used data from a German cost of blindness study by Lafuma et al. (2006) [22]. Total costs were corrected with income losses, in order to guarantee a consistent assessment. Total costs were adjusted to 2008 prices using the consumer price index.

Table 7.9 shows an overview of indirect costs included in the model.

7.3 Cost of Illness in Germany

This section summarises the results of the cost-of-illness study. Total costs include all costs (direct medical and indirect cost) in relation to the CMV infection. Costs were discounted at 5%.

7.3.1 Total Societal Costs

Every year in Germany, an estimated 6500 children are born with congenital cytomegalovirus (CMV) infection, of which 1500 are primary infected. Of the latter around 495 suffered from symptoms at birth. The remaining number of children is without symptoms but remote damages. An estimated number of 36 children die from primary CMV infection. 460 children suffer from permanent disabilities such as hearing or vision loss or mental retardation. 5000 children from seropositive women are asymptomatic at birth, and in 750 cases remote damages appear; approximately three died. Altogether around 1200 children (primary infected and from seropositive women) remain with permanent disabilities. These 1200 disabled children cause major socio-economic impact, since they need lifetime care and treatments.

Table 7.9 Overview of indirect costs

Indirect cost	Avg. cost per year in €	Avg. duration in years	Source
Cost of schools			
– School for blind people	10,333	10	[7]; own calculations
– School for deaf people	10,333	20	[7]
– School for mild handicapped people	6126	15	[23]
– School for severe handicapped people	44,835	20	[23]
– School for mild deaf people	2583	20	[7]; own calculations
– Average wage special mobile teacher	37,277	10	Information of Ministry of Internal Affairs 2009
Cost of nursing home	37,483	20	[24]
Employment of the mother (forgone earnings, changing work situation)			
– Impact – child < 6 years	3418.58	Per year	[21]; own calculations
– Impact – child between 6 and 10 years	2084.36	Per year	[21]; own calculations
– Impact – child between 11 and 18 years	672.34	Per year	[21]; own calculations
Nursing leave (parents)		20 days/year	
– Nursing leave – child < 6 years	923.92	Per year	[21]; own calculations
– Nursing l. – child between 6 and 10 years	1319.47	Per year	[21]; own calculations
– Nursing l. – child between 11 and 18 years	1761.84	Per year	[21]; own calculations
Productivity loss due to death (mean male and female gross salary)	42,419	From age of majority up to the average retirement age/year	[14]
Cost of blindness (from the age of 18 years on)	9497	Per year	[22]; own calculations

Table 7.10 depicts the total cost of CMV infection in Germany per child and for society as a whole, differentiated according to the groups of children affected. Total costs depend on the number of children affected and the cost per child.

From the societal perspective, the overall average cost per patient over lifetime was 766,444€ (2.97 m€ undiscounted). Indirect costs represented 92% of the total costs. Considering the indirect/direct costs, the major cost driver was costs for special schools, followed by lost human capital for dead children, nursing homes and work absenteeism. Costs for the whole society amount to 242.91m€ (940.77 m€ undiscounted) per year.

Table 7.10 Total costs of CMV infection

Total costs	€/per child	€/all affected children
Children with symptoms at birth and w/o remote damages ($n = 257$)	766,878	197,394,287
Children with symptoms at birth and remote damages ($n = 238$)	1,245,069	295,828,484
Children without symptoms at birth and remote damages ($n = 186$)	478,192	88,907,812
Children of seropositive women and remote damages ($n = 750$)	478,192	358,643,855
Total costs ($n = 1431$)	2,968,331	940,774,438
Total costs discounted	766,444	242,914,561

Quelle: IPF own calculations

Table 7.11 Direct costs

Direct cost	€/per child	€/all children affected
Children with symptoms at birth and w/o remote damages	68,379	17,600,874
Children with symptoms at birth and remote damages	99,613	23,668,004
Children without symptoms at birth and remote damages	31,233	5,807,061
Children of seropositive women and remote damages	31,233	23,425,012
Total direct costs	230,459	70,500,951
Total direct costs discounted	59,506	18,203,840

Quelle: IPF own calculations

7.3.1.1 Direct Cost

Table 7.11 depicts the direct costs of the CMV model, for each group of children.

A further differentiation is that of the settings: inpatient and ambulant. Results are shown in Table 7.12.

The main proportion, namely, 85% of direct costs, arises in the ambulant or outpatient setting. Inpatient costs occur mostly in the first year after birth.

7.3.1.2 Indirect Costs

Indirect costs are the overwhelming cost component and exceed direct costs by far. Ninety-two percent of total costs are indirectly disease associated. Table 7.13 shows the indirect cost of the CMV model, differentiated according to the groups of children affected per child and for the society.

A further differentiation has to deserve the following components: absenteeism, nursing leave, human capital of dead people, cost of blindness, schools and nursing homes. The indirect costs are distributed as shown in Fig. 7.2.

Out of the indirect costs, the major cost drivers were costs for special schools, followed by lost human capital for dead children, nursing homes and work absenteeism.

Table 7.12 Direct costs of the settings

Direct costs of different settings	€/child inpatient	€/all affected children inpatient
Children with symptoms at birth and w/o remote damages	11,527	2,967,141
Children with symptoms at birth and remote damages	15,629	3,713,518
Children without symptoms at birth and remote damages	4102	762,651
Children of seropositive women and remote damages	4102	3,076,446
Inpatient costs	35,360	10,519,756
Inpatient costs discounted	**9130**	**2,716,275**
	€/child ambulant	€/all affected children ambulant
Children with symptoms at birth and w/o remote damages	56,852	14,633,732
Children with symptoms at birth and remote damages	83,984	19,954,486
Children without symptoms at birth and remote damages	27,131	5,044,410
Children of seropositive women and remote damages	27,131	20,348,566
Outpatient costs	195,098	59,981,194
Outpatient costs discounted	**50,376**	**15,487,565**

Source: IPF own calculations

Table 7.13 Indirect costs

Indirect cost	€/per child	€/all affected children
Children with symptoms at birth and w/o remote damages	698,498	179,793,414
Children with symptoms at birth and remote damages	1,145,457	272,160,480
Children without symptoms at birth and remote damages	446,958	83,100,751
Children of seropositive women and remote damages	446,958	335,218,843
Total indirect costs	2,737,872	870,273,488
Total indirect costs discounted	706,938	224,710,721

Source: IPF own calculations

7.3.2 Sensitivity Analysis

Since economic data are frequently incomplete and associated with uncertainty, assumptions need to be made regarding the values for certain parameters. Therefore, following the primary case analysis, the results were tested for stability using a deterministic sensitivity analysis. The following variations were calculated:

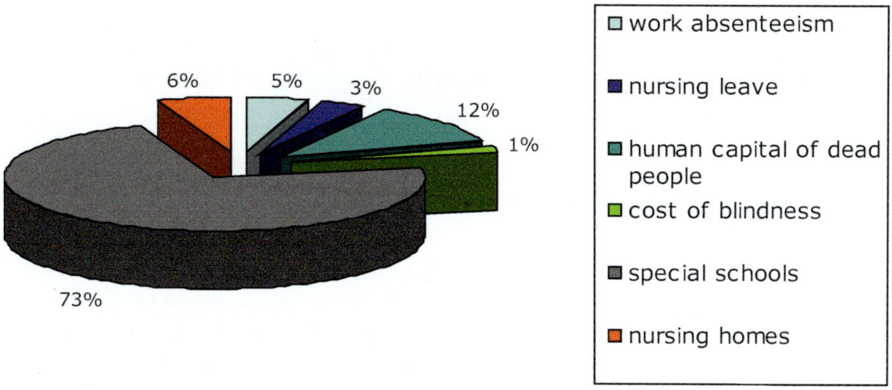

Fig. 7.2 Distribution of indirect costs. Source: IPF own calculations

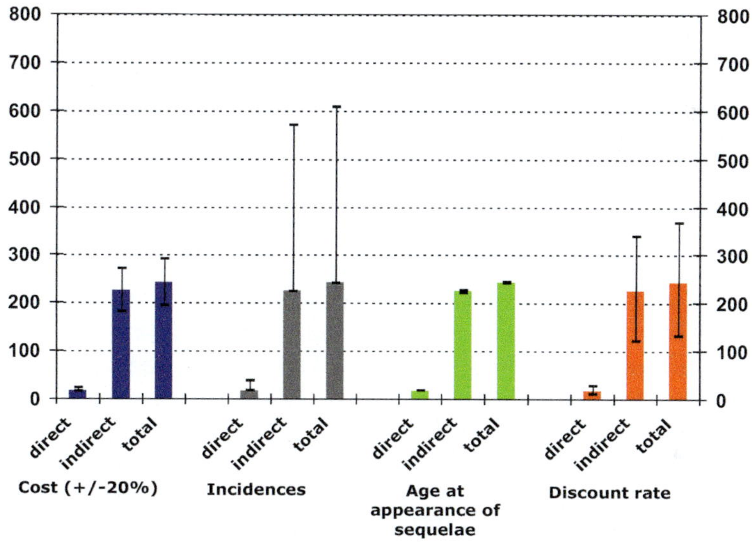

Fig. 7.3 Results after variation. Source: IPF own calculations

- Variation 1: cost (not discounted) ±20%
- Variation 2: incidences of symptoms (incidences for the minimum and maximum values are derived from literature)
- Variation 3: age at appearance of sequelae → min: 6 months; max: 5 years
- Variation 4: discount rate → min: 3%; max: 10% according the German Recommendations on Health Economic Evaluation

The results are presented in Fig. 7.3.

The factors with the greatest influence on costs were the incidence rates of sequelae, with a possible impact of double costs. The incidence rates used for the sensitivity analysis were derived from a literature search. This result reflects the importance of reducing the occurrence of sequelae through preventive strategies. The results of the sensitivity analysis moreover show the conservative approach of the cost-of-illness study.

7.3.3 Impact Through Prevention

Commonly, prevention strategies are classified into three alternatives: primary, secondary and tertiary prevention. Primary prevention tries to avoid the occurrence of infection, i.e. hygiene measures and change of behaviour. Secondary prevention strategies mean early detection, with the aim of stopping progression of infection and disease. In the case of symptomatic disease, tertiary prevention strategies try to prevent the appearance of severe sequelae after infection. Prenatal primary and secondary screening strategies as well as postnatal secondary and tertiary screening strategies are an important public health question, but have not yet been implemented by any European country [2]. To discuss the issue more rationally, economic studies are necessary.

The aim of this section is to show the budget impact of CMV secondary prevention – prenatal screening and prenatal management – in relation to total cost of illness of CMV infection. Different secondary prenatal screening strategies exist; we analysed the following one:

- Serological testing of all pregnant women with a CMV IgG and IgM test ($n = 700{,}000$) according to the diagnostic algorithm for CMV [25, 26]. CMV IgG ELISA is an accurate serologic method to detect CMV IgG antibody for identification of CMV infection. The clinical sensitivity exceeds 99% [27].
- Follow-up tests in seronegative women (in Q2 and Q3) ($n = 350{,}000$) (expert opinion).
- An IgG avidity assay is used to distinguish between primary and recurrent CMV infection (all women that were CMV IgM positive) ($n = 40{,}000$) [25].
- Second follow-up test of IgG, IgM and IgG avidity of approximately $n = 30{,}000$ of women that were one-time IgM positive.
- Prevention with CMV immunoglobulin Cytotect® (n = 3500). According to Negro et al. (2007), the application of Cytotect® leads to a significant reduction of transmission of foetuses from 50% to 3% [28].

Table 7.14 depicts the calculation of prevention cost of CMV in Germany.

Total cost for diagnosis and prevention is 61.41 m€, whereas costs for testing represent 42.48 m€ and the application of CMV immunoglobulin 18.93 m€. Resource use for secondary prenatal strategy takes place in the first year considered; therefore, discounting is not needed. CMV testing and administration of CMV-specific immunoglobulin reduce the total societal cost due to CMV infection to 163 m€ (455 m€ undiscounted). This was associated with a significant lower risk of congenital CMV infection (minus 640 infants). Thus, the budget impact amounts to 80 m€ (486 m€). Every Euro spent for CMV prevention leads to a saving of 1.30 €

Table 7.14 Prevention and impact on budget

Prevention	Number of tests	€
No. of CMV IgG and IgM first investigation	700,000	21,000,000
Follow-up tests of IgG and IgM in Q2 and Q3 of all seronegative (M- G-) women (approximately 88.6%)	310,000	18,600,000
First follow-up test of women with M+ (IgG, IgM and avidity test)	40,000	1,644,000
Second follow-up test of IgG, IgM and avidity test of women that were one-time IgM positive	30,000	1,233,000
Total CMV IgG, IgM and IgG avidity tests	2,230,000	42,477,000
Prevention with CMV immunoglobulin	3500	18,928,000
Total cost for diagnosis and prevention		61,405,000
Cost per CMV IgG test (€)	15	
Cost per CMV IgM test (€)	15	
Cost per CMV IgG avidity test (€)	11.1[a]	
Cost per prevention (2 × 2 ml/kg bw) (€)	5408[b]	
	Not discounted	Discounted
CMV total cost with prevention	**454,976,690 €**	**163,027,972 €**
Budget impact	485,797,748 €	79,886,589€
Every 1 € spent for CMV prevention leads to a saving of	**7.91**	**1.30**

[a]Source: EBM
[b]Assumption: Infusion in ambulant setting, four times
[c]Cost of medication: average value of hospital cost (=€ 520)
Source: Munro et al. (2005), Lazzarotto et al. (2008); IPF own calculations

(7.91 € undiscounted). The definite conclusion based on this calculation is that a secondary prenatal strategy being highly cost-effective leads to cost savings for the whole society, reduces significantly the number of children with sequelae and decreases the disease burden for parents and their children.

7.4 Discussion

CMV infection is the most frequent congenital infection and the major cause of neurological and sensory impairment in children. Both primary and recurrent infection due to this virus can result in foetal infection. The most severe congenital disease occurs following a primary maternal infection during pregnancy. In Germany each year, an estimated 6500 children are born with congenital CMV infection, causing an estimated 40 death and leaving approximately 1200 infants with permanent disability. The disease burden due to CMV infection concerning epidemiology and disability and information relating to the actual costs are not well-documented. The objective of this study was to estimate the total economic impact on German society based on the CMV infection related to direct and indirect costs applying the societal point of view. Costs for the whole society amount to 242.91 m€. These costs arise due to CMV infection every year.

Information about resource use and clinical data in children with CMV infection and sequelae was collected by means of literature and experts. The used bottom-up approach allowed us to estimate costs, e.g. for specific groups of children with and without symptoms at birth and children with or without remote damages, more accurately than it would have been possible with a top-down approach. This method of resource use calculation may have been led to an over- or underestimation of used resources. Unit costs were valuated with social insurance prices and fees. In countries with a social insurance system, in other words, a "fee for service system", tariffs underestimate costs, because they may include other incentives. As a consequence we performed a sensitivity analysis to check possible cost implications when increasing/decreasing the direct cost by 20%. The range was 14.56 m€ to 18.2 m€ for societal direct costs. It can be stated generally that a slight under- or overestimation of direct costs will have relatively little effect as they represent only 8% of the total costs.

In a burden of illness assessment, indirect costs must be included. The present study identifies high indirect costs. Ninety-two percent of total costs represent indirect costs, because indirect costs over the lifetime are incurred by parents and their affected children. However, estimating indirect costs is a methodological problem as they cannot be measured directly. We used the most commonly applied human capital approach although it has limitations regarding the economic assumptions it is based upon [29, 30]. Indirect costs are influenced by the assumed discount rate for future costs occurring through productivity loss. We used the recommended discount rate of 5% [13]. Applying a lower discount rate of 3% or a higher rate of 10% would substantially influence indirect costs (range 120.24 m€ to 338.69 m€). Furthermore, the main cost drivers were the incidence rates of sequelae. More disabled children lead to a significant higher productivity loss and nursing effort. However, literature reports are controversial regarding incidence rates for, e.g. petechiae, hearing loss, microcephalus, mental retardation, convulsions, etc. Depending on the used incidence rates, indirect costs for society may reach 569 m€ for German society. We chose a conservative approach for the cost-of-illness study and excluded outliers.

Based on the cost-of-illness results, we conclude that the estimated 1200 infants with permanent disability, infected within 1 year, cause a disease burden of 243 m€ (130 m€–607 m€) to the German society.

CMV is a prime target for prevention, not only because of its disease burden but also because there are ways to reduce viral transmission [1]. The implementation of any prevention strategy of CMV infection should be based on reliable estimates of epidemiology and costs, e.g. the incidence of CMV infection in various countries, the positive and the negative predictive values of prenatal diagnosis, the efficacy of prenatal treatment and the proportion of infants born with symptoms and permanent disability. The financial implications of serology testing and management of infected foetuses should also be evaluated. This present cost-of-illness study shows explicit for the first time that routine screening of all pregnant women results in a positive budget impact for Germany. Total costs for diagnosis and prevention are 61.41 m€, whereas costs for IgG, IgM and IgG avidity testing represent 42.48 m€ and the application of CMV immunoglobulin 18.93 m€. We used the study from Negro et al. (2005) to report the treatment effect of hyperimmune IgG against CMV. The finding however remains controversial as the study was lacking a strict randomised protocol [2] and only 31 women received hyperimmune IgG [28]. However, at present, other studies are not available, and a publication bias favouring cases in which hyperimmune globulin treatment had a positive effect cannot be excluded [2].

CMV IgG testing and administration of CMV-specific immunoglobulin reduces the total societal costs due to CMV infection from 242.91 m€ to 163 m€ and this every year. This was associated with a significant lower risk of congenital CMV infection (minus 640 infants). Thus the budget impact amounts to 80 m€ every year. Every Euro spent for CMV prevention leads to a saving of 1.30€. Apart from costs, a reduced number of infected children is associated with a significant quality of life gain. Health-related quality of life is the part of people's quality of life that health and healthcare can potentially influence, e.g. with a prevention strategy. Health-related quality of life (HRQoL) is an increasingly important outcome measure in healthcare, reflecting the transition of disease burden from CMV infection to permanent disability. Its measurement is important for rational public health policy, as it allows direct comparison between different conditions and interventions using quality-adjusted life-years (QALYs). Regarding CMV related sequelae utility values are: utility value of patients with bilateral visual loss range from 0.2 to 0.8 [31, 32], that at mild mental retardation values 0.64 [33]. In addition to QALYs the Global Burden of Disease Study has calculated disability weights as life lost by virtue of being in states of poor health or disability: mild mental retardation weights 0.36, deafness 0.33 and blindness 0.62.

The definite conclusion based on this analysis is that a secondary prenatal strategy is highly cost effective, leads to cost savings for the whole society, significantly reduces the number of children with sequelae and decreases the disease burden for children and their parents.

Addendum

Gabriele Halwachs-Baumann

In January 2018 a cost-of-illness study was published by Korndewal et al. [1], calculating the costs of congenital CMV. As a result it was shown, that the average healthcare costs of children with congenital CMV in the first 6 years of life are much higher than that of children without congenital CMV (€ 6113 vs. € 3570, converted to 2018 US dollars i.e. $ 7327 vs. $ 4279). For those children with long-term impairments the healthcare costs are twice as high in children with congenital CMV (€ 17,205, i.e. $ 20,624) compared with children without congenital CMV (€8332, i.e. $ 9987). This emphasizes the evidence that congenital CMV is not only a massive health problem, but also (for those who believe in an economic view of the world) an enormous economic problem. Additionally there are several reasons to presume that the actual difference in health care costs between the congenital CMV-positive and congenital CMV-negative children is larger than found in this study, since children who died of congenital CMV within the first 5 years of life were not included, and the healthcare costs were estimated only up to 6 years of age [1]. Calculating the cost for the whole life this would multiply the direct cost for congenital CMV infection by ten, as shown in the chapter before. So reducing the number and the severity of congenital CMV infection will definitely save money. Nevertheless, the amount of reduced costs depends on the choosen defence strategy.

To fight congenital CMV infection different approaches are under discussion:

1. Vaccination as it is performed to eradicate congenital rubella syndrome.
2. Education on hygienic procedures to avoid infection during pregnancy
3. Screening pregnant women and prophylaxis/therapy with hyperimmune globulin in the case of primary CMV infection
4. Screening newborns and treatment with antivirals

Although it sounds easy, a lot of questions arise. In the case of vaccination despite the issue which vaccine should be used, it is important to decide the group of people who should be vaccinated. For rubella four different strategies are described [2]: in the United States vaccination of all children to create herd immunity and later, revaccinating all young adult women is performed. The program of the United Kingdom includes vaccination of teenage girls and sero-negative women plus contraception for three months after vaccination. The Swedish program consists of vaccination in early childhood and re-vaccination of all teenagers. In Iceland a selective vaccination involving puerperal women as well as all women of child bearing age who are willing to use contraceptives for three months is performed. For rubella it was shown that vaccination to prevent congenital rubella syndrome is more cost-beneficial than vaccination to interrupt rubella transmission [2]. Furthermore, since vaccine prices have fallen over the year, it was mentioned that blind vaccination has become more favorable compared to targeted vaccination.

For congenital CMV infection vaccinating all adolescent females prior to their first pregnancy would cost $ 32.3 million dollars less than not vaccinating. This was true under the presumption that vaccine efficacy against disease is at least 61%. When vaccine efficacy against disease was less than 61%, not vaccinating would became the preferred strategy because it was less expensive than vaccinating, without substantial changes in clinical benefits to the population [3]. In the paper from N'Diaye et al [4] also the vaccinating strategy was evaluated. They compared their current practice, which consists of hygiene counseling, with routine vaccination of all adolescent women aged 14 years old, and screening and vaccination of the seronegative women as third strategy. The results were similar to those found by Dempsey et al: Systematic vaccination of adolescent girls was found to be the most efficient strategy to prevent maternal seroconversons. As a limitation seroprevalence was mentioned. If the seroprevalence was more than 62% screening and vaccination of seronegative would become the most efficient strategy [4].

Vaccinating strategies to prevent congenital CMV infection must be viewed under the perception, that the burden of CMV transmission and disease following non-primary infection in pregnancy may be higher than previously anticipated [5]. The fact that preexisting immunity of the mother is an incomplete protective shield against transmission is known for a long time. Nevertheless, transmission rate in primary infections is said to be 30% opposed to a rate between 1 and 2% in non-primary infections [5]. So it seems to be worthwhile to evaluate vaccination strategies not only with the goal to prevent transmission in seronegative women, but also to enlarge immunological defense against CMV transmission in seropositive women. That means that trying to stimulate immune responses similar to those seen in natural infection may not suffice to protect all women against CMV transmission to their offspring [5].

One of the most economic intervention strategies to prevent infection of women is an educational approach. As it is known the shedding rate of healthy young children is much higher than that of seropositive healthy adults [6]. Thus toddlers are likely transmitters of CMV to their mothers, or other persons taking care of these children for example in a crèche or a kindergarten. Giving women instructions about protective behaviors and risky behaviors to avoid, seroconversion rate can be halved [7]. Since the percentage of people who have heard of congenital CMV is alarmingly low (7 % of men, 13 % of women), educational programs would be an effective way to reduce CMV transmission to pregnant women [8, 9, 10]. Although compared to other prevention strategies information and education is the least effective strategy, it is also the least costly [4], with no side-effects and no investments but time. So this should be the least to fight against congenital CMV infection.

As discussed in the study above prophylaxis with hyperimmuneglobulin is another option to prevent congenital CMV infection. Universal screening for primary maternal CMV infection with intention to treat with CMV i.v. immune globuline was shown to be the most cost-effective strategy compared to selective screening strategies [11, 12]. However, if immunoglobulin treatment achieves less than a 47% reduction, other strategies would be more cost-effective.

To evaluate the efficacy of CMV hyperimmunglobulin administration during pregnancy it is important to differentiate whether this intervention was to prevent transplacental transmission from mother to child, or it was given as therapeutic application to reduce symptoms in the yet infected unborn. Since it is crucial to find the point in time at which transmission has already occurred, results on the efficacy of hyperimmunglobulin administration are sometimes contradictory. We can hope that ongoing studies will elucidate these problems.

One strategy to fight the harm caused by intrauterine CMV infection which is quite well investigated is the antiviral intervention after birth. Cost effectiveness of newborn screening was evaluated under a wide range of assumptions. Most studies focused on the prevention or at least improvement of hearing loss. Since hearing loss after congenital infection is a slow progressive disease, antiviral treatment is an effective intervention. These clinical experiences are substantiated by pathophysiological investigations [13]. The estimated total lifetime costs of severe or profound hearing loss are $ 280,000 per child, plus an estimated productivity loss of $ 926,000, resulting in approximately $ 1.2 million total costs [14], which incur if nothing is done. Comparing these costs with those arising by screening and therapy programs, every economist must rise up his hand to vote for programs reducing the problems induced by congenital CMV. So compared to the above mentioned cost of ignorance, the estimated costs of identifying a case of congenital CMV-related hearing loss by targeted congenital CMV screening using salivary swabs vary between £ 9224 and £ 5413 (converted to 2018 US dollars i.e. $ 12,390 and $ 7,273). The costs of 'protecting' a case of congenital CMV related hearing loss by antiviral treatment vary between £ 19,601 and £ 11,502 (converted to 2018 US dollars i.e. $ 26,330 and $ 15,450). These are costs comparable to other screening and interventions programs used for the detection of phenylkentonuria or cystic fibrosis [15]. Just focused on the mitigation of hearing loss by antiviral treatment public savings will offset the public costs incurred by screening and treatment if just one infant per year benefits from this program [16]. This is accompanied by costs of $ 2000–$ 10,000 for identifying one case of congenital CMV infection among all infants born in the United States by universal screening and $ 566–$ 2832 by targeted screening. Just focused on identifying hearing loss due to congenital CMV detecting one case costs $ 27,460 by universal screening or $ 975 by targeted screening. Also in this study universal as well as targeted screening reduce total costs under most assumptions [14]. It was even shown that net savings from universal screening were greater than those from targeted screening, although screening costs are higher.

Taking together it can be said that whatever the program is you choose to reduce the number of children congenitally infected with CMV or to mitigate symptoms due to congenital CMV infection—there is a benefit not only from a medical and humanitarian point of view but also from an economical point of view. The most expensive action is to be in denial and to do nothing.

References

1. Korndewal MJ, Weltevrede M, van den Akker-van Marle ME, Oudesluys-Murphy AM, de Melker HE, Vossen ACTM (2018) Healthcare costs attributable to congenital cytomegalovirus infection. Arch Dis Child 103(5):452–457
2. Babigumira JB, Morgan I, Levin A (2013) Health economics of rubella: a systematic review to assess the value of rubella vaccination. BMC Public Health 13:406–418
3. Dempsey AF, Pangborn HM, Prosser LA (2012) Cost-effectiveness of routine vaccination of adolescent females against cytomegalovirus. Vaccine 30 (27):4060–4066
4. N'Diaye DS, Launay O, Picone O, et al (2018) Cost-effectiveness of vaccination against cytomegalovirus (CMV) in adolescent girls to prevent infections in pregnant women living in France. Vaccine 36(10):1285–1296
5. Plachter B (2016) Prospects of a vaccine for the prevention of congenital cytomegalovirus disease. Med Microbiol Immunol 205:537–547
6. Stowell JD, Mask K, Amin M, et al (2014) Cross-sectional study of cytomegalovirus shedding and immunological markers among seropositive children and their mothers. BMC Infect Dis 14:568–579
7. Adler SP, Finney JW, Manganello AM, Best AM (1996) Prevention of child-to-mother transmission of cytomegalovirus by changing behaviors: a randomized controlled trial. Pediatr Infect Dis J 15(3):240–246

8. Cannon MJ, Westbrook K, Levis D, Schleiss MR, Thackerey R, Pass RF (2012) Awareness of and behaviors related to child-to-mother transmission of cytomegalovirus. Prev Med 54(5):351–357
9. Picone O, Vauloup-Fellous C, Cordier A-G, et al (2009) A 2-year study on cytomegalovirus infection during pregnancy in a French hospital. BJOG 116:818–823
10. Vauloup-Fellous C, Picone O, Cordier AG, et al (2009) Does hygiene counseling have an impact on the rate of CMV primary infection during pregnancy? Results of a 3-year prospective study in a French hospital. J Clin Virol 46(Suppl 4):S49–S53
11. Cahill AG, Odibo AO, Stamilio DM, Macones GA (2009) Screening and treating for primary cytomegalovirus infection in pregnancy: where do we stand? A decision-analytic and economic analysis. Am J Obstet Gynecol 201:466 e1–e7
12. Johnson JM, Anderson BL (2013) Cytomegalovirus: Should we screen pregnant women for primary infection? Am J Perinatol 30:121–124
13. Halwachs-Baumann G. (2016) Congenital cytomegalovirus infection and hearing impairment. Clin Res Infect Dis 3(2):1029–1032
14. Gantt S, Dionne F, Kozak FK, et al (2016) Cost-effectiveness of universal and targeted newborn screening for congenital cytomegalovirus infection. JAMA Pediatrics 170(12):1173–1180
15. Williams EJ, Gray J, Luck S, Atkinson C, et al (2015) First estimates of the potential cost and cost saving of protecting childhood hearing from damage caused by congenital CMV infection. Arch Dis Child Fetal Neonatal Ed 100: F501–F506
16. Bergevin A, Zick CD, McVicar SB, Park AH. (2015) Cost-benefit analysis of targeted hearing directed early testing for congenital cytomegalovirus infection. Int J Pediatr Otorhinolaryngol; 79(12):2090–2093

References

1. Cannon MJ, Finn Davis K (2005) Washing our hands of the congenital cytomegalovirus disease epidemic. BMC Public Health 5:70
2. Ludwig A, Hengel H (2009) Epidemiological impact and disease burden of congenital cytomegalovirus infection in Europe. Euro Surveill 14(9):26–32
3. Porath A, McNutt RA, Smiley LM et al (1990 Jan–Feb) Effectiveness and cost benefit of a proposed live cytomegalovirus vaccine in the prevention of congenital disease. Rev Infect Dis 12(1):31–40
4. Gazelle GS, McMahon PM, Siebert U et al (2005 May) Cost-effectiveness analysis in the assessment of diagnostic imaging technologies. Radiology 235(2):361–370
5. Akobundu E, Ju J, Blatt L et al (2006) Cost-of-illness studies – A review of current methods. Pharmacoeconomics 24(9):869–890
6. Azam AZ, Vial Y, Fawer CL, Zufferey J, Hohlfeld P (2001) Prenatal diagnosis of congenital cytomegalovirus infection. Obstet Gynecol 97(3):443–448
7. Halwachs-Baumann G, Genser B (2003) Die konnatale Zytomegalievirusinfektion Epidemiologie – Diagnose – Therapie. Springer, Wien

8. Halwachs-Baumann G., Ludwig A., Hengel H., Cytomegalie-virus (CMV) – Infektionen in der Schwangerschaft. www.dgk.de, o.J.
9. Ornoy A, Diav-Citrin O (2006) Fetal effects of primary and secondary cytomegalovirus infection in pregnancy. Reprod Toxicol 21:399–409
10. Dollard S, Grosse S, Ross D (2007) New estimates of the prevalence of neurological and sensory sequelae and mortality associated with congenital cytomegalovirus infection. Rev Med Virol 17
11. Ramsay M, Miller E, Peckham C (1991) Outcome of confirmed symptomatic congenital cytomegalovirus infection. Arch Dis Child 66
12. Schöffski O, von der Schulenburg Graf JM (2008) Gesundheitsökonomische Evaluation. Wiener Medizinische Wochenschrift 159(5–6):160–168
13. von der Schulenburg Graf JM, Greiner W, Jost F et al (2007) Deutsche Empfehlungen zur gesundheitsökonomischen Evaluation – dritte und aktualisierte Fassung des Hannoveraner Konsens. Gesundh ökon Qual Manag 12. https://doi.org/10.1055/s-2007-963505
14. Statistisches Bundesamt Deutschland http://www.destatis.de/jetspeed/portal/cms/Sites/destatis/Internet/DE/Navigation/Navigationsknoten__Startseite1.psml
15. WHO Global Burden of Disease, http://www.who.int/topics/global_burden_of_disease/en/
16. Institut für Gesundheitsökonomik München (2008) Bundeseinheitlicher Basisfallwert für Krankenhausleistungen und seine Konsequenzen: ein falscher Weg aus ordnungspolitischer Sicht.
17. AOK (2008) Gesundheitskasse für Niedersachsen-Leistungen Hörgeräte. www.aok.de
18. Sohlbach I., Burgdörfer J., Lang J. (2008) Blindheit und Sehbehinderung. www.polizei-projekte.nrw.de
19. Leitlinien der Gesellschaft für Neonatologie u Pädiatrische Intensivmedizin Zerebrale Anfälle beim Neugeborenen, 2004
20. Leitlinien der Gesellschaft für Neuropädiatrie, Wahrnehmungsstörungen, 2001
21. Lange K, Danne T, Kordonouri O et al (2004) Diabetesmanifestation im Kindesalter: Alltagsbelastungen und berufliche Entwicklung der Eltern. Deutsche Medizinische Wochenschrift 129
22. Lafuma A, Brezin A, Lopatriello S et al (2006) Evaluation of non-medical costs associated with visual impairment in four European countries. Pharmacoeconomics 24(2)
23. Preuss-Lausitz U (2004) Zur Frage der Kosten gemeinsamer schulischer Bildung. www.ewi.tu belin.de/files/resourcesmodule/@random435c8d75c8731/1131958614_Kosten11_05.ppt
24. AOK (2009) allg. Pflegesatz, Vollstationäre Pflege, www.aok-pflegenavigator.de
25. Munro SC, Hall B, Whybin LR et al (2005) Diagnosis of and screening for cytomegalovirus infection in pregnant women. Journal of Clinical Microbiology 43(9):4713–4718
26. Lazzarotto T, Guerra B, Lanari M et al (2008) New advances in the diagnosis of congenital cytomegalovirus infection. J Clin Virol 41
27. Curdt I, Herzogenrath J, Bernhardt S, Braun HB, Eichler R, Maine GT, Hausmann M, Stricker RT, Stricker RN, Lazzarotto T, Christ H (2006) Preliminary evaluation of the Abbott ARCHITECT anti cytomegalovirus IgG, IgM and IgG avidity assays linked by an automated reflex algorithm. American Association for Clinical Chemistry Annual Meeting, Chicago
28. Nigro G, Adler SP, La Torre R, Best M (2005) Passive immunization during pregnancy for congenital cytomegalovirus infection. N Engl J Med 353:1350–1362
29. Drummond MF (1986) Studies in economic appraisal in health care, vol 2. Oxford University Press, Oxford
30. Drummond MF (1992) Cost of illness studies: a major headache? Pharmacoeconomics 2:1–4
31. Brown GC, Brown MM, Sharma S, Brown HC (1998) Patient perceptions of quality-of-life associated with bilateral visual loss. Int Ophthalmol 22(5):307–312
32. Weintraub WS (2003) Cardiovascular health care economics. Humana Press, Totowa, NJ
33. Insinga RP, Laessig RH, Hoffman GL (2002) Newborn screening with tandem mass spectrometry: examining its cost-effectiveness in the Wisconsin Newborn Screening Panel. *J Pediatr.* 141:524–531

Printed by Printforce, the Netherlands